W9-BLW-218

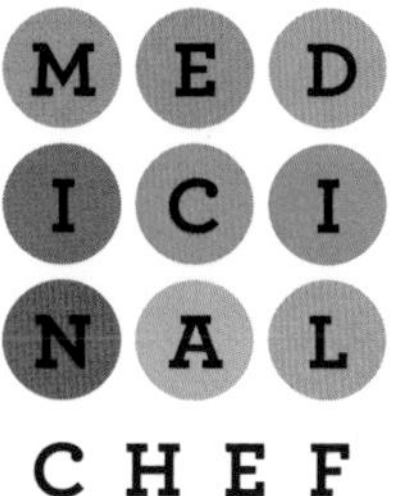
MED
ICI
NAL
CHEF

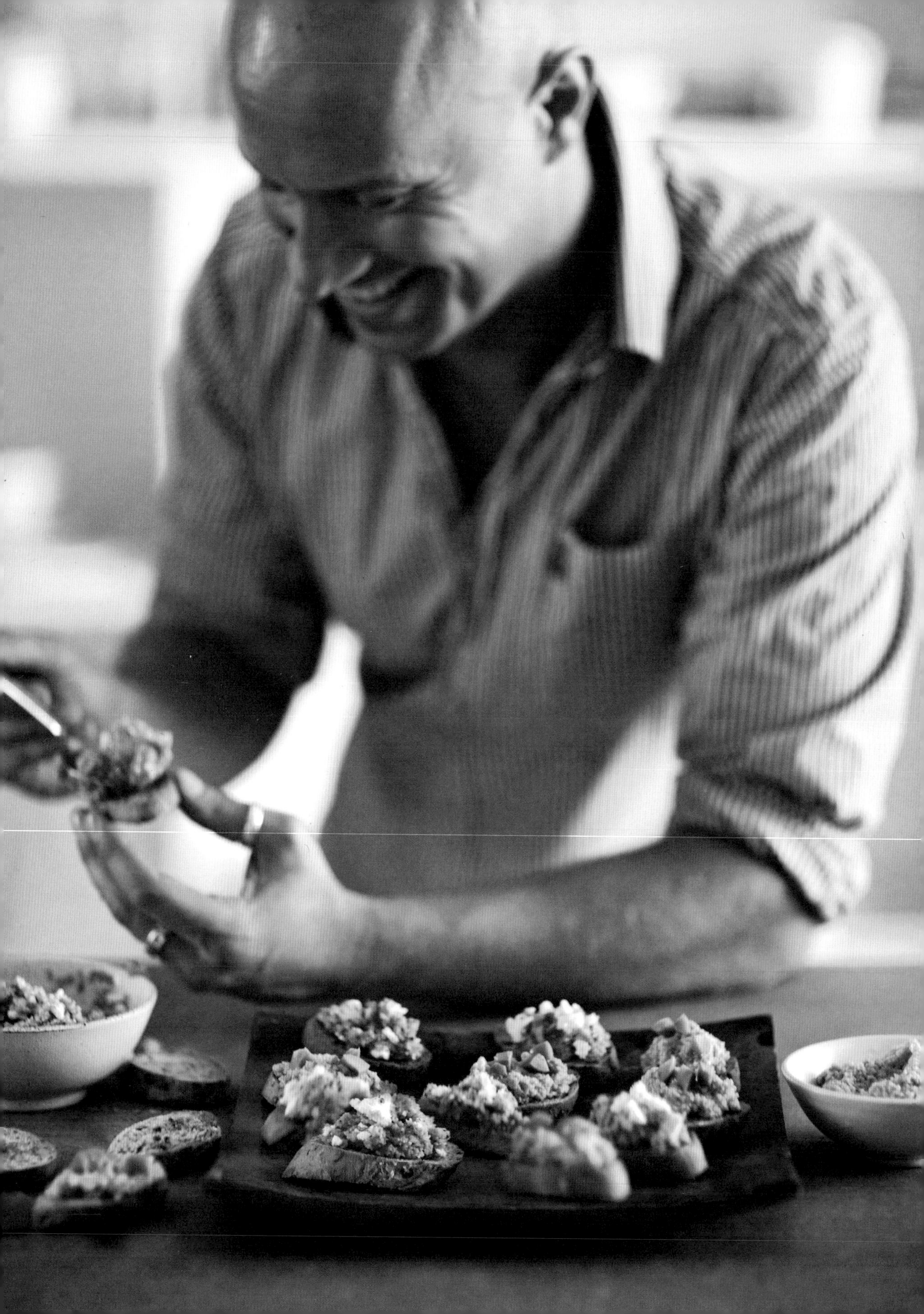

DALE PINNOCK

The MEDICINAL CHEF

Eat Your Way to Better Health

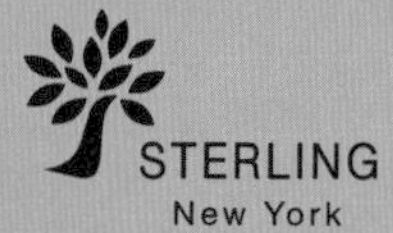

CONDITIONS

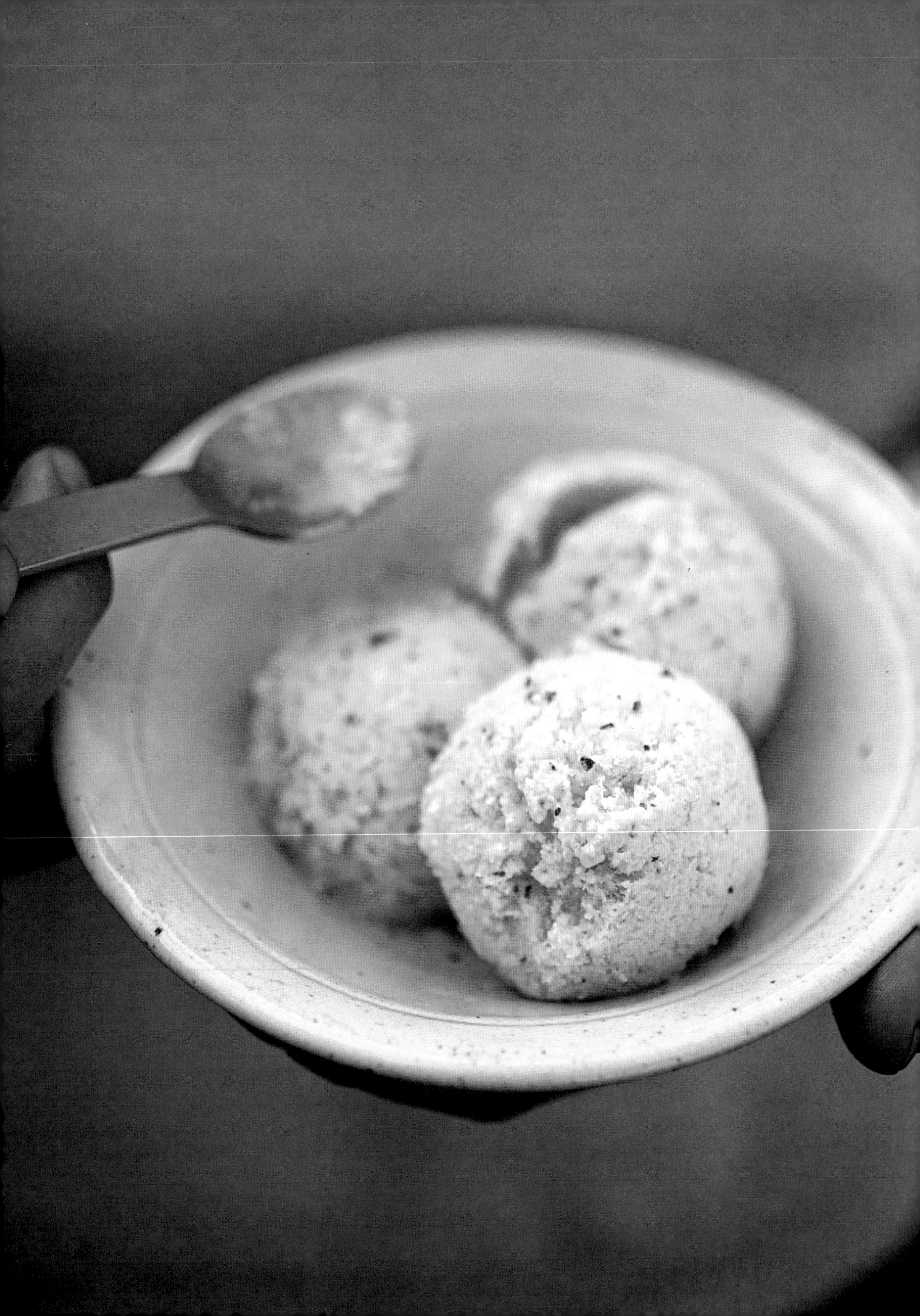

FOOD AS MEDICINE

Throughout history, many medical systems have recognized the important role that food can play in the healing process. Traditional Chinese medicine and Indian Ayurvedic medicine are two wonderful examples of how observations about the interactions between food and our bodies can be pooled and used as a therapeutic tool. For a long time in the West, as the modern medical establishment came into its own, the importance of this knowledge has been forgotten. When we are sick we go straight to the doctor. Our treatment is out of our hands, and we rely solely on the professionals to return us to good health. For many years, the only real study of nutrition was into its role as a food source. We knew that a lack of certain nutrients could cause deficiency diseases, such as the role of vitamin C in rickets and scurvy, but that was as far as it went.

A few decades ago, however, interest in nutrition and its potential role in health care began to increase once more. Health food stores began popping up in every mall. Books started appearing on the subject, some of which are now cult classics, and all manner of weird, wacky, and wonderful diets and health care regimes started appearing. The scientific establishment began to question, and even oppose, aspects of this movement—sometimes with good reason, but occasionally to such an extent that anyone discussing the connections between nutrition and health was at risk of being dismissed as a charlatan.

THE EVIDENCE

In the meantime, though, much research was being done in the area. Some were large-scale, population-based research studies, such as the National Health and Nutrition Examination Survey, which has been assessing the health and nutrition of people across the US since the early 1960s; and the British National Diet and Nutrition Survey, a wide-ranging survey of the nutrition in the UK Others were intervention studies, testing the effects of specific diets and nutrients on health and disease. From all of this, we started to get a better understanding about what was really going on. We quickly began to learn what was having an effect and what wasn't—and we are still only at the very beginning of this process. It gave rise to a strong evidence base for food as a medicine in its own right, and also finally put to bed some of the strange diets and oddball myths. As a result, what was once often deemed quackery is now considered a valid part of the health care picture.

HOW CAN FOOD HELP US BECOME HEALTHIER?

Many of us view food simply as the fuel we need to consume to keep us going. Things like carbohydrates and proteins—the macronutrients—are just that, providing energy and materials for growth and repair. But the thing is that food is so much more. As well as the macronutrients, there are the micronutrients: the vitamins, minerals, trace elements, and essential fatty acids. These are the keys that allow chemical events to take place in the body. Zinc, for example, is used to regulate our white blood cells and the way the brain uses and responds to its own chemistry; it even creates proteins that regulate inflammation. Essential fatty acids are the building blocks for hormones and a whole group of communication molecules that work to regulate pain and inflammation. The B vitamins turn food into energy, and magnesium is essential for more than 1,000 chemical reactions in the body. So it's clear that getting enough vitamins and minerals will have a huge impact on our daily health.

Things get really exciting, however, when we start to look at the compounds in many ingredients that aren't strictly nutrients, since none of them are essential for health, but which can deliver medicinal effects in their own right. Enter the phytonutrients. These are chemicals in plants such as color pigments, hormones and structural compounds. They are starting to be widely researched and are proving to have some wondrous effects. Chemicals in cherries can help beat insomnia. Chocolate can lower blood pressure. Red wine can protect us from heart disease. And that is just the beginning! When we put these things together, it becomes clear that what we eat can have a very profound effect upon our capacity to get better.

MY PHILOSOPHY

I have no belief or interest in the concept of alternative medicine. I used to, but times have changed as I have evolved personally and professionally. I am not dismissive of natural therapies, but I'd like to move away from the idea of them being an "alternative" or replacement for "conventional" medicine, which is rather unhelpful. As far as I am concerned, there are many elements to consider when it comes to health; it's not simply a case of conventional versus alternative. If somebody is sick and they need pharmacological drugs, then they need drugs. End of story. But that doesn't mean there isn't also much they can do for themselves by making changes to their diet and lifestyle.

Let's use high blood pressure as an example. This causes a real risk of serious cardiovascular disease, since the pressure will increase the risk of damage to the inner lining of the blood vessels, which can lead to heart disease. Medication that decreases the pressure and takes the burden off the cardiovascular system may save lives. But at the same time, it's also important to make diet and lifestyle changes. Intakes of sodium and bad saturated fats need to be reduced, and food's glycemic index (the increase in blood sugar levels after eating it), needs to be considered. And other nutrients can counter some of the changes taking place inside the body. A group of compounds called flavonoids, found in green tea, onions, and dark chocolate, can increase the chemicals that widen the blood vessels and reduce blood pressure. Eating more omega-3 fatty acids will naturally decrease levels of the chemicals that tighten the blood vessels. All these things have been well researched, documented, and understood, so we can see that there is a valid place for the use of diet in the management of high blood pressure, as well as many other conditions.

In my view, the problem arises when we have a polarized, all-or-nothing approach to treatment. Just diet, or just medication, in isolation will only have a narrow spectrum of benefit. If we bring the two approaches together, the therapeutic spectrum is much broader. When we understand that there is more than one thing we can do to get well, we are in a better position to return to good health.

MY ROLE AS THE MEDICINAL CHEF

That's where I come in: to look at the science about which foods can be useful for certain physiological changes and diseases, assess what dietary changes we can easily make, and use my culinary skills to create practical, delicious dishes that everyone can cook and enjoy in their day-to-day life. I'm fascinated by the science of nutritional medicine, and I've also been a serious food lover for most of my life—I've even worked as a chef. I've always loved new, exciting, delicious, and most of all, real food. I want to show you that proper food that will improve your health isn't sawdust-like muesli, mung beans, or rabbit food. We can take pleasure from our food, and at the same time know it will help with our health.

Eating this way can be an exciting culinary journey, and you don't have to sacrifice flavor, style, or enjoyment. Dishes such as the Greek pita pizzas (page 70), Tuna steaks with sweet potato wedges and greens (page

118), or the Mint chocolate no-cheese cake (page 148), are true stars—they're packed with flavor and won't feel like anything less than a treat. The other thing you'll notice is that all the recipes are simple, quick, and easy. This is about healthy cooking in the real world. Many of the recipes are one-pot wonders, they're all easy to shop for at the supermarket, or grocery store and don't need any specialist equipment. Many are ready in less than half an hour. And, most importantly, all of them are tasty!

HOW TO USE THIS BOOK

Every recipe includes symbols to indicate which of the body systems and specific conditions it can help, so you can look out for the recipes that will benefit you most. If you're just after a dish that will give your body a boost, everything in here is good for you! The recipes are divided into chapters according to the kind of thing you want to eat. For a quick lunch, turn to Light Bites (page 60); to find ideas for sharing a feast with friends, turn to Small Plates, Sides & Sharing (page 74); for something quick to eat after work, turn to Quick Main Courses (page 102); if you want something a bit more ambitious. turn to Weekend Main Courses (page 122). There's a good-for-you option every time you need it!

To find out what you can eat to help with specific medical conditions, turn to Conditions (page 164), where you'll find details of the 30 ailments in which food has been most convincingly identified as having a significant role to play. For each condition, you'll also find a list of the most effective recipes to try, and the ingredients to look out for. If you're interested in finding out more about the effects of individual foods, turn to Ingredients (opposite), where there's a directory of the main ingredients that have been shown to have health benefits. If you want to find out more about the evidence of links between food and health, have a look at Further Reading (page 191).

So, that's what *The Medicinal Chef* is about: not alternatives or miracle cures, but simple and enjoyable tools that will help us all move toward better health—with a full stomach and a smile on our face.

INGREDIENTS

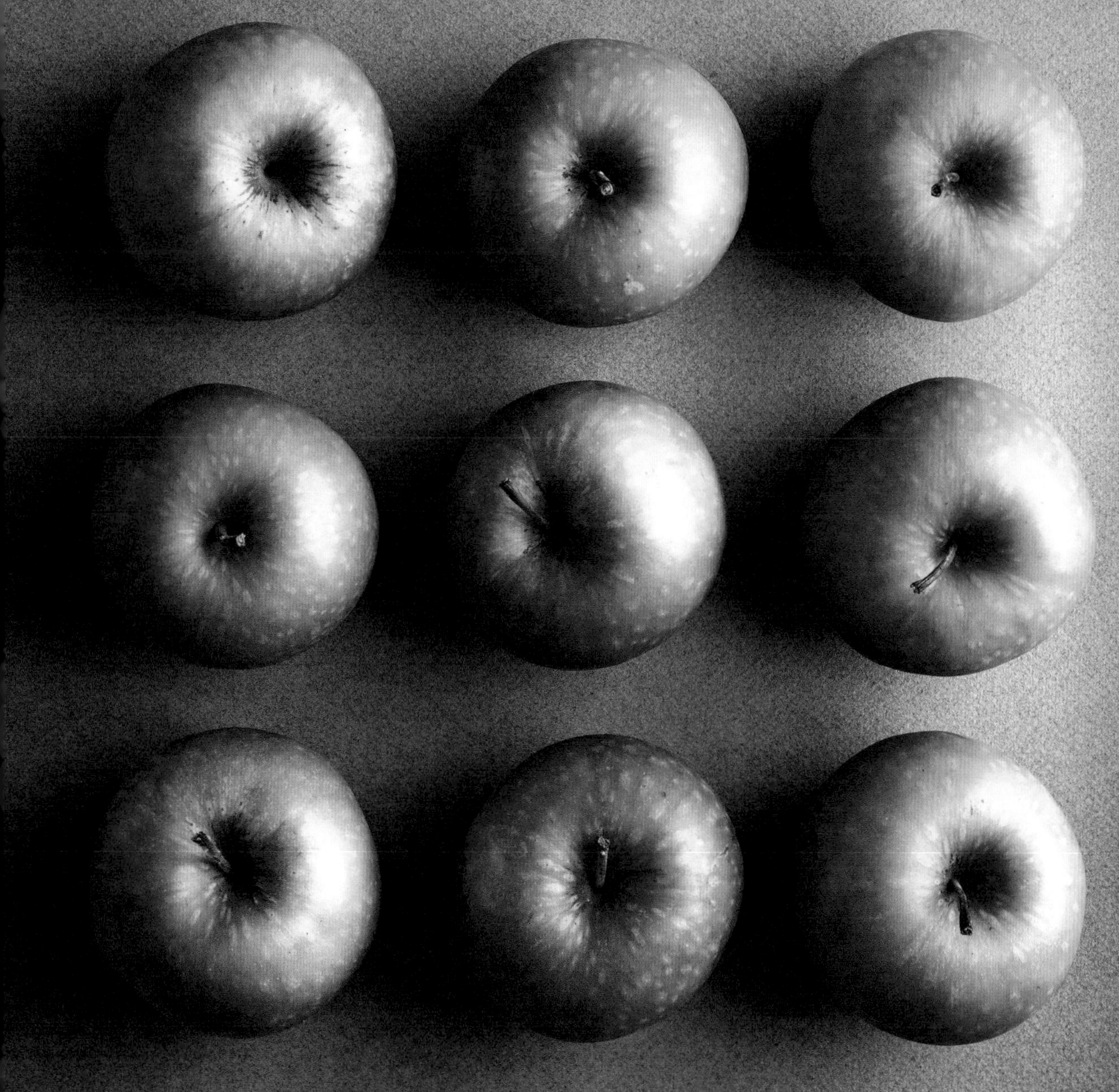

FRUIT

APPLES

High cholesterol
Apples contain a unique type of soluble fiber called pectin. This fiber can help carry cholesterol out of the digestive system. When the liver makes cholesterol, a very high proportion of it is sent into the digestive tract, where it is absorbed into the bloodstream. If we can reduce this, we can reduce cholesterol levels. This is how cholesterol-lowering drinks work.

Asthma
Some research has indicated that a chemical called phloridzin in apples can help to reduce localized inflammation in the lungs, for example in asthma. There are also very high levels of a compound called quercetin in apples, which has a natural, subtle antihistamine activity.

BANANAS

Insomnia
Bananas are very high in an amino acid called tryptophan, which is converted into the neurotransmitter serotonin in the brain. This neurotransmitter helps regulate sleep patterns.

High blood pressure
Bananas are very high in potassium. This helps buffer the effects of salt on the body, which include contraction of the blood vessels and increased fluid retention, all of which cause an increase in blood pressure. Sodium-potassium balance is an important part of managing blood pressure. Of course, it's not as simple as just eating a banana, and then everything is all right; it's just a great example of a good food to include in your diet.

BLUEBERRIES

Heart & circulation
A lot of what you hear about the amazing health properties of blueberries is exaggerated, but they are high in the antioxidant compounds anthocyanidins. These are the compounds that give them their deep purple color, and have been shown to cause relaxation of blood vessels, protect blood vessel walls against damage, and even reduce cholesterol slightly.

Eye health
Some of the antioxidants in blueberries have been clinically tested, and have shown potential benefit in cases of macular degeneration (loss of vision in the center of the visual field) and cataracts. They are not a cure, but may help with prevention.

CHERRIES

Anti-inflammatory
Cherries are bursting with compounds called anthocyanins, which give them their deep ruby red color. They are known to work in a similar way to some prescription anti-inflammatories (although they are not an alternative) by blocking the activity of certain enzymes that stimulate inflammation. This can help with many conditions, including gout, arthritis, and joint pain.

Insomnia
Montmorency cherries in particular are known to be very high in a compound called melatonin, which is also secreted in the brain as a sleep-inducing hormone. Many clinical studies have shown that eating fresh cherries or small servings of cherry juice can effectively induce sleep.

Gout
The anthocyanins unique to cherries have also been shown to be effective against gout. This painful condition is caused by uric acid crystals accumulating in joints, where they can put pressure upon soft structures within the joint. Cherry anthocyanins actually inhibit the action of an enzyme called xanthine oxidase, which produces uric acid.

CRANBERRIES

Urinary system health
Cranberries have a longstanding reputation as a powerful remedy for treating urinary tract infections such as cystitis, and rightly so. Most urinary tract infections are caused by *E. coli* bacteria. When they embed themselves in the wall of the urethra, the immune system responds and the urinary tract becomes inflamed. This is what causes the symptoms.

Cranberries are very high in compounds called proanthocyanidins, which prevent *E. coli* from attaching to the urethral wall.

DATES

High cholesterol
Dates are very high in a type of soluble fiber called beta glucan. Many clinical trials have shown beta glucan to be effective at lowering cholesterol. It does this by binding to cholesterol in the digestive tract, and carrying it away through the bowels.

Constipation
Beta glucan is wonderful for softening the stool and stimulating mild contraction of the gut wall, enabling better elimination.

GOJI BERRIES

Immune system health
No longer difficult to find in most health stores, goji berries contain a very special type of large sugar molecule called polysaccharides. These sugars have been shown to increase the production of white blood cells, the army of the immune system. This makes goji berries a useful ingredient during colds and flu, and for keeping the immune system strong at other times, too.

Healthy eyes
Goji berries are packed with two key antioxidants, lutein and zeaxanthin, both of which help protect the macular in the retina of the eye from free-radical damage. High-level consumption has been linked to protection from eye damage and improvements in eyesight.

GRAPES

High blood pressure
Grapes contain two clinically tested, powerful compounds that can affect blood pressure. The first is the deep purple pigment from a group of compounds called oligomeric proantocyanidins (say that quickly and I'll give you $5!). The second is a compound called resveratrol. This works in a similar way, and they complement each others' action. They increase the production of compounds naturally released by the cells that line the blood vessels, which cause the muscles in the blood vessel walls to relax, making the vessels widen. The wider the vessel, the lower the pressure.

High cholesterol
Grapes don't seem to contain any cholesterol-lowering compounds per se, but they do contain compounds that reduce the oxidation of cholesterol. This highly reactive chemical process causes notable damage to blood vessel walls, and is one of the reasons that reducing cholesterol is a good idea.

LEMONS & LIMES

Colds & flu
The first good thing about citrus fruits is that they are packed with vitamin C. This is vital for immune function, as it allows white blood cells to attack bugs more ferociously. Lemons and limes are also rich in a compound called kaempferol, which has notable antibiotic properties. These have been demonstrated epidemiologically (by studies of general health patterns), as well as clinically.

MANGOS

Skin health
The bright orange flesh of the mango is produced by a high concentration of beta-carotene, a fat-soluble antioxidant that can quickly move into the skin and protect it from free radical damage that can lead to wrinkles and premature aging. Beta-carotene also has anti-inflammatory activity, too.

Digestive system health
There is a group of enzymes in mango that are proteolytic, which means they help the body to digest proteins more effectively. If you are going to eat mango for this reason, though, I would recommend eating it before a meal rather than after it, since fruit on top of a meal can actually cause digestive discomfort.

PAPAYAS

Bloating & indigestion
Papaya contains a very powerful enzyme called papain, which is known to be very beneficial for digestion. It is especially useful for indigestion caused by eating too much high-protein food—such as an enormous steak! Papain is also useful for easing bloating by improving the digestion and breakdown of food components.

PINEAPPLES

Arthritis
Pineapple contains a very powerful enzyme called bromelain, which actually blocks certain aspects of the

inflammatory response from occurring. Pineapple has a great track record for benefiting many painful inflammatory conditions. However, most of the bromelain is found in the tougher inner core of the pineapple, the bit that most of us throw away; in very ripe pineapples, though, it is often edible.

Digestive system health
Bromelain is also thought to be a useful digestive aid, especially for high-protein foods.

VEGETABLES

ARTICHOKES

Diabetes
Artichokes are very high in a type of sugar called inulin, which has been shown to stabilize blood sugar levels, as it slows down the release of glucose from other foods, thus reducing blood sugar spikes.

Liver & digestive system health
Artichokes contain a compound called caffeoylquinic acid, which is thought to protect the liver from inflammatory damage and increase the production and flow of bile. This offers protection from gallstones and relief from constipation. Bile is basically the body's own natural laxative.

High cholesterol
Some trials using artichoke extract showed reductions in bad (LDL) cholesterol. This may in part be due to its effect on bile flow, since bile is one of the main ways in which cholesterol is transported from the liver.

ASPARAGUS

Urinary system health
Asparagus has been a traditional medicine in Asia for centuries. It contains a unique compound called asparagine, which increases urinary output. This can be very useful in conditions such as high blood pressure and fluid retention.

Anti-inflammatory
A chemical in asparagus called racemofuran has been identified as having mild anti-inflammatory activity.

AVOCADOS

High cholesterol
Avocados are very high in a fatty acid called oleic acid, also found in olive oil, which many trials have shown causes a reduction in bad (LDL) cholesterol, and a subtle increase of good (HDL) cholesterol.

Skin health
They are also very high in the fat-soluble antioxidant vitamin E. This helps protect skin cell membranes from damage, and can be an important part of a natural skincare regime.

Heart & circulation
The high vitamin E content of avocados makes them a wonderful food for heart health. Vitamin E is a natural anticoagulant, meaning it reduces blood clotting activity and may offer protective benefit against heart attack and stroke.

BEANS

High cholesterol
All beans are naturally very high in fiber, which is of immense benefit to the cardiovascular system. As we know, fiber has an important "cleansing" effect on digestive health and ensures that things move along adequately. This helps the cardiovascular system as it helps get rid of cholesterol. When the body manufactures cholesterol in the liver, some of it gets absorbed there and then, while the rest moves, via bile, from the liver into the digestive tract, where more gets absorbed. A good intake of fiber can actually reduce the absorption of some of this cholesterol, helping keep cholesterol levels in check.

Digestive system health
Beans, like all high-fiber foods, are a must for healthy digestion. Fiber swells within the digestive tract, increasing the bulk of the digestive contents. When this occurs, specialized stretch receptors detect the increase in volume and stimulate the contraction of the muscles that line the gut wall. This rhythmical contraction, known as peristalsis, is what keeps everything moving through the gut as it should.

Reproductive system health
Some types of beans, such as soybeans and chickpeas, are rich in a group of compounds called isoflavones. These compounds are similar in structure to estrogen and can actually bind to estrogen receptors in susceptible tissues. It is important to know that although

they bind to estrogen receptors, there is no evidence that they stimulate an estrogenic effect.

Some hormonal issues, such as the menopause and PMS, involve symptoms that result from changes in estrogen levels. This can either cause tissues to go into overdrive because too much estrogen is present, or create a reaction because estrogen levels have dropped considerably. When there is excess estrogen, it is thought that isoflavones can bind to the estrogen receptors, and stop the real estrogen from overstimulating the tissues. On the other hand, when there is insufficient estrogen and the receptors are deprived, the binding of isoflavones to the receptors can reduce some of the withdrawal symptoms that are experienced.

BROCCOLI

Cancer prevention
I'm always wary of claims that one individual ingredient or lifestyle change can cause cancer or prevent it, and the same is true here. However, broccoli does contain some chemical compounds that, in laboratory studies at least, seem to offer some prevention against cancerous changes in cells. The compounds indole-3-carbinole and sulfuraphane are the most widely studied. This doesn't mean you can smoke 20 a day if you eat broccoli, though—it's just an interesting insight into the powerful effects foods can have.

Stomach ulcers
Some research suggests that sulfuraphane may help to kill the bacteria *H. pylori*, which is involved in stomach ulcers.

BUTTERNUT SQUASH

Acne & eczema
The color of the beautiful bright-orange flesh comes from a group of compounds called carotenoids, fat-soluble antioxidants that will move into the lower layers of the skin quite quickly. Their localized anti-inflammatory activity can reduce the redness of lesions such as eczema and acne. They also help protect collagen fibers from damage, and so are a great anti-aging ingredient.

Heart & circulation
Carotenoids can reduce the oxidation of fatty compounds such as bad (LDL) cholesterol, which can damage the blood vessels. These damaged areas get plugged with cholesterol and scar tissue, and heart disease ensues. Reducing the oxidation gives some reduction in risk.

CABBAGE

Cellular spring cleaning
I don't believe in faddy detox diets, but the body does detoxify itself naturally. Every second of every day, every cell is breaking down and removing waste products. Cabbages, like all members of the *Brassica* family, are packed with compounds such as isothiocyanates (try saying that backward!), which actually increase the levels of some of the enzymes involved in the process.

Heart & circulation
Some of the phytochemical compounds in cabbage are known to reduce the levels of a substance called homocysteine, which has been linked with increased risk of heart disease.

CARROTS

Skin health
The vivid orange color of carrots is thanks to beta-carotene. This compound naturally diffuses into fatty tissues such as those in the skin, where it can offer localized antioxidant protection and anti-inflammatory activity. This is ideal for conditions such as acne and eczema.

Eye health
The old saying that carrots can help you see in the dark isn't true. I bet that comes as a shock! It was actually part of wartime propaganda. That said, carrots do offer some benefits to eye health, thanks to the beta-carotene. This fat-soluble nutrient can accumulate in the eyes and offer protection against free-radical damage, which may help protect against cataracts.

CELERY

Pain reduction
Despite its innocent appearance, celery packs a powerful medicinal punch. It contains a powerful compound called 3-n-butylphthalide (3NB for short), which is an effective pain killer. It's not going to be replacing morphine any time soon, but it's an easy-to-incorporate ingredient and

anecdotal evidence has shown it to be effective for conditions like arthritis, sprains, and injuries. Isn't salad fun?

Urinary system health
Celery contains a complex cocktail of components that give it a potent diuretic activity. Firstly, it contains a group of compounds called coumarins. These help give it its distinctive smell, and are the same compounds that give a freshly mowed lawn its fragrant aroma. They also increase urinary output. Add to this very high levels of potassium, and you have a notable increase in urinary output. Try drinking some celery juice and see what happens! This makes it useful for urinary tract infections and even high blood pressure.

EDAMAME BEANS

Reproductive system health
Edamame, or soybeans, are one of the richest sources of isoflavones on the planet. These are estrogen-like compounds that can bind to estrogen receptors and have been shown to offer some benefits in issues such as menopause and endometriosis.

High cholesterol
Regular consumption of soybeans has been shown to lower bad (LDL) cholesterol.

EGGPLANTS

Nervous system health
A compound called nasunin, found in the skin of the eggplant, has recently been identified, which is thought to protect the fatty coating of nerve cells from damage.

Constipation
Eggplants are high in fiber, helping to soften the stool and move things along nicely.

FAVA BEANS

Digestive system health, heart & circulation
Like all beans, fava beans are very high in fiber, which delivers benefits to two body systems. Firstly, high-fiber foods benefit digestion by ensuring regularity. The fiber attracts water and swells in the digestive tract, which strengthens the natural contractions of the gut wall (known as peristalsis), and keeps everything moving along nicely. The fiber content also helps the cardiovascular system, as it helps to carry cholesterol out of the gut, and can reduce overall cholesterol levels. They are also very rich in potassium, which helps reduce blood pressure.

FENNEL

Digestive system health
The oils that give fennel its distinctive flavor are known to ease cramps and spasm in the digestive tract, so it's ideal for gripey digestive discomfort. The very same oils also help dispel gas and wind and ease bloating.

JERUSALEM ARTICHOKES

Digestive system health
Jerusalem artichokes are like dynamite for the digestion, and for the uninitiated, your first experience with them may be somewhat explosive! Do persist, though, as it will quickly settle down. They are very high in a compound called fructo-oligosaccharide (FOS), and another one called inulin, which are both prebiotic compounds, in other words a food source for the "good" bacteria in the gut. When these bacteria feed on them, they start to reproduce, making their numbers stronger. These good bacteria help regulate many aspects of digestive health, from improving transit to repairing the gut wall, and even manufacturing certain nutrients.

KALE

Osteoporosis
Kale is high in calcium, and is also rich in phosphorous. This ratio supports bone health: if phosphorous levels are too high and calcium levels too low, it increases the risk of osteoporosis.

Muscular cramps
Its dark green color means that kale is incredibly rich in chlorophyll. Chlorophyll contains magnesium, and calcium and magnesium work in tandem in muscle tissue. Calcium causes muscle to contract, whereas magnesium causes it to relax. Any kind of muscle cramp or spasm will always benefit from additional magnesium.

LEEKS

Digestive system health
Like all of the *Allium* family (such as onions, chives, and garlic), leeks are very high in the prebiotic compound inulin.

This feeds the good bacteria in the gut, enabling them to reproduce, strengthening the colony, and improving digestive function.

Heart & circulation
The *Allium* family contains high levels of sulfur-based compounds, which are known to reduce blood clotting. These compounds also seem to have a favorable effect upon cholesterol levels.

OLIVES

Digestive system health
One of the most noticeable thing about olives is their bitter flavor. This is key to how they can help digestion. When we taste something bitter, a nervous reflex takes place, and as a result of this, the gall bladder contracts and releases a squirt of bile. Bile is essential for fat digestion, and also works as the body's own built-in laxative. This reflex also increases production of gastric juices, so protein digestion will be improved slightly.

Heart & circulation
The fatty acids in olive oil have been shown to be beneficial for the health of the heart. They can increase the levels of good (HDL) cholesterol, and decrease the bad. Oleic acid in olive oil also seems to have a beneficial effect on blood pressure.

ONIONS

Allergies
Onions are very high in a compound called quercetin, which has a mild but effective antihistamine activity. Allergies involve a localized release of histamine by white blood cells, which causes the inflammation and irritation.

Asthma
Onions, particularly the red variety, contain several compounds which can reduce inflammation, particularly in the respiratory tract, so they may be useful for asthmatics.

Digestive system health
Onions, like all of the *Allium* family, are rich in a compound called inulin, which is a potent prebiotic. This will increase the numbers of "good" bacteria, which regulate virtually every aspect of digestive health.

PARSNIPS

Digestive system health
Parsnips contain a special type of sugar called inulin, which is responsible for the sweet flavor. It is a potent prebiotic, which means it is a good food source for the good bacteria that lives in the gut. When these bacteria reproduce and increase in numbers, they also secrete compounds that help repair the gut lining and regulate movement through the gut.

PEA SHOOTS

Immune system health
Move over citrus fruits—pea shoots are a seriously good source of vitamin C. And, since these little shoots are eaten raw and when very fresh, their nutrient levels are superior. Not only are they a great hit of sunshine, they are also an excellent way to get that vital vitamin C hit during the winter months.

Protein generation
All sprouting seeds are dense in all the essential amino acids our bodies need to make protein. These nutrients are much more concentrated in plants during the early stages of their growth cycle, so sprouts are full of them. We don't necessarily need to consume protein to make protein; what we need are essential amino acids (the ones our bodies cannot make themselves and must be obtained from the diet), which will then be sent to the liver to be used to make human proteins.

PEPPERS

Skin health
Red and orange bell peppers are packed with two very powerful fat-soluble antioxidant compounds: carotenoids and flavonoids, both of which contribute to the vivid colors. They rapidly diffuse into the fatty layer of the skin, where the collagen and elastin fibers are at their most dense, and help protect collagen from damage. This can reduce the wrinkling and skin aging. They can also deliver some localized anti-inflammatory activity, and may be useful for eczema and acne.

Heart & circulation
Flavonoids are also beneficial for the health of the blood vessels, making the inner lining of vessels more resilient to damage. It is damage to this inner lining that helps cause buildup of plaques in the cardiovascular system.

POTATOES

High blood pressure
The humble potato, although it can be a bit of a starch bomb, has been found to contain kukoamine, a compound once only known to exist in a few obscure Chinese herbs. It doesn't occur in many plants, and has been shown to cause a mild reduction in blood pressure. How it works isn't clear yet, but it represents a glimmer of hope for potato lovers. A word of caution, however: too much of any starchy food isn't good for the heart at all, as they can upset blood sugar levels quite rapidly.

RED BEETS

High blood pressure
Red beets have been the focus of a great deal of clinical research in recent years. One of the areas that has attracted a lot of attention is the effect beets have on blood pressure. Beets are very high in natural nitrates, a type of mineral salt. This is converted by the body into nitric oxide, which is naturally produced to regulate blood pressure. Nitric oxide causes the muscles in the blood vessel walls to relax, which widens the vessels, and in turn reduces blood pressure. Some small-scale studies have confirmed this effect. This doesn't mean you can throw your medicine in the garbage and eat red beets all day, though—it just highlights a powerful ingredient we can consume more of to benefit our health.

Liver health
Several studies have shown that betacyanin, the purple color pigment in red beets, can have a beneficial effect on liver function. It is known to increase the level and activity of detoxification enzymes found in the liver, mainly the potent glutathione peroxidase, which is involved in breaking down and removing alcohol from the liver. Bacon sandwich the morning after? Nah. Bring on the red beet juice!

RED CABBAGE

Anti-inflammatory
The deep purple color is delivered by a powerful group of antioxidants called anthocyanins. These deliver a reasonable amount of anti-inflammatory activity, especially for the digestive tract and cardiovascular system. They also help reduce some of the chemicals that actually trigger inflammation in the first place.

Heart & circulation
Anthocyanins have been shown to stimulate the cells that line the inner surface of blood vessels to secrete a chemical called nitric oxide, which relaxes the muscles in the blood vessel walls. This in turn lowers blood pressure. The effect is temporary, but it is one of the ingredients you can add to your diet to help manage high blood pressure.

SHIITAKE MUSHROOMS

Immune system health
Shiitake mushrooms are one among a few varieties of mushroom that contain a powerful, unique sugar called polysaccharides. There are many of these in nature, but the type found in shiitake mushrooms are beta-glucans, and these have been researched globally for more than 40 years. One area in which there is the strongest evidence is the effect they have upon the immune system. They have been shown to cause an increase in the production of white blood cells (our immune system's army), and their response to pathogens or damaged cells. Just a small amount of these compounds daily can really give the immune system a bit of a boost.

High cholesterol
A decade or two ago, a substance in shiitake mushrooms called eritadenine was discovered. It was found that this compound could lower bad (LDL) cholesterol, while improving levels of the good (HDL) cholesterol. It is believed that it does it by influencing the way in which the liver produces cholesterol in the first place.

SPINACH

Skin health
Not only is it a good source of vitamin C, protein, and iron, spinach is also packed with the potent fat-soluble antioxidant beta-carotene, which can naturally and rapidly diffuse into the lower, fatty layer of the skin, where it can protect collagen and elastin fibers from damage.

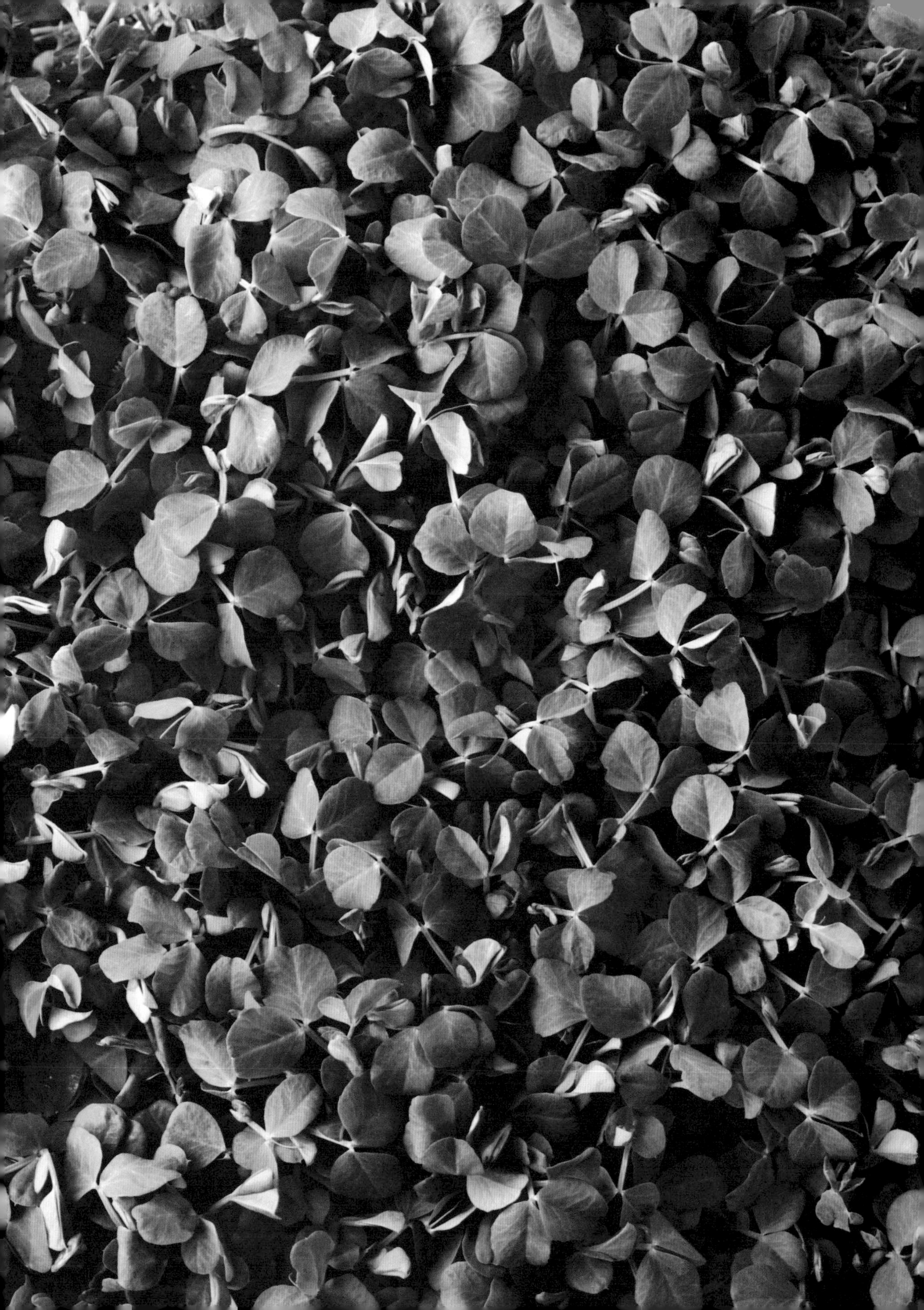

SPIRULINA

Skin health & neurological system
Spirulina is an extremely nutritious algae that is very high in B vitamins. These are vital for turning food into energy, maintaining a healthy skin, and regulating many activities in the central nervous system.

Natural energy boost
Spirulina is an amazing vegetarian protein source: it's 60–70% protein, and provides the full spectrum of essential amino acids we need every day. With B-vitamin and protein levels like these, spirulina is a great natural energy booster.

SWEET POTATOES

Immune system health
Sweet potatoes contain a unique type of storage protein used by the plant as a food source during various stages of its growth cycle. Research carried out in China has shown that this protein may stimulate the production of white blood cells, possibly helping with immunity.

Skin health
Sweet potatoes are also rich in beta-carotene, the substance that gives them their bright orange color. This can offer significant antioxidant protection for the skin, and some anti-inflammatory action, too.

TOMATOES

Heart & circulation
Tomatoes are an important component of the well-documented health benefits provided by the Mediterranean diet. They are packed with two important antioxidant nutrients: vitamin C and lycopene. Lycopene is a carotenoid compound responsible for much of their red color. These are important to heart health because they reduce lipid peroxidation, a type of naturally occurring damage to dietary fats. These can cause damage to the blood vessel walls, which may then set the stage for heart disease.

Prostate health
There has been a great deal of research on the link between lycopene and prostate health, but the evidence is mixed. There is, however, some evidence to suggest that populations that consume high levels of lycopene tend to have fewer prostate-related health problems.

DAIRY & FISH

ANCHOVIES

Heart & circulation
The high level of vital omega-3 fatty acids in anchovies help maintain healthy cholesterol levels and offer protection against damage to the blood vessel walls caused by inflammation, which starts the heart disease process.

Asthma & eczema
Omega-3 fats also help the body create its own natural anti-inflammatory compounds, which in turn can reduce inflammation. That's why these fats are vital in managing all inflammatory conditions, such as asthma, eczema, and arthritis.

Bones & joints
Anchovies have a wonderful mineral content, so I would recommend them for conditions such as osteoporosis, as they are very high in calcium, magnesium, phosphorous, and vitamin D. All of these are key players in maintaining bone mineral density.

EGGS

Heart & circulation
Eggs have been much maligned for their cholesterol content, but actually they are pretty much the best protein source on the planet, for the simple reason that the protein is 100% usable. And eggs are also very rich in betaine, a nutrient known to reduce homocysteine, which is a potent compound linked to increased risk of heart disease.

Nervous system health
Eggs are also very rich in choline, which helps to maintain the structural integrity of the fatty structures surrounding our nerve cells. This makes them helpful for any nervous disorder, from the perspective of basic maintenance if nothing else.

FETA CHEESE

Digestive system health
Good-quality feta is made from sheep's milk, which is often far better tolerated by the digestive tract and is less likely to cause the stomach upsets that can be quite common with cow's milk cheese.

GOAT CHEESE

Digestive system health
The properties of goat cheese are the same as feta, with an even higher level of tolerance for those who are usually intolerant to dairy produce, so they can be even easier on the digestion.

HERRING

Arthritis, eczema & asthma
Like all oily fish, herring is packed with omega-3 fatty acids that help the body produce its own powerful anti-inflammatory compounds. These make all oily fish important for tackling inflammatory conditions.

Heart & circulation
Omega-3 fatty acids are vital for heart health. Firstly, they protect the blood vessels from inflammatory damage. Secondly, they help decrease levels of bad (LDL) cholesterol, and increase levels of good (HDL) cholesterol. They also play a role in reducing blood clotting.

Rickets & osteoporosis
Oily fish such as herring are packed with vitamin D, one of the most commonly deficient nutrients. Vitamin D is vital for facilitating the absorption of calcium, and a deficiency of it in a developing child may cause rickets, while deficiency in adulthood can increase and exacerbate osteoporosis.

MACKEREL

Arthritis, eczema & asthma
Mackerel is incredibly high in vital omega-3 fatty acids. These help the body to produce its own built-in anti-inflammatory compounds. This makes it great for inflammatory conditions.
Heart & circulation
The omega-3 fatty acids have a very favorable effect upon cholesterol levels, and can also protect blood vessel walls from inflammatory damage.

Osteoporosis & rickets
Oily fish, and especially mackerel, are very high in vitamin D, which is vital for the proper utilization of calcium in the body. The main source of vitamin D for humans is the conversion of cholesterol into vitamin D upon exposure to UV radiation—in other words, the sun! Thankfully, there are also a few food sources, and oily fish are top of the list.

SALMON

Heart & circulation
Salmon is packed with omega-3 fatty acids, those all-important good fats. These help maintain healthy cholesterol levels and protect the blood vessels from inflammatory damage, which can be the first step in the process that later leads to heart attacks. Omega 3 is also beneficial for the rate and extent to which blood clots.

Arthritis, asthma & eczema
Omega-3 fatty acids are very powerful anti-inflammatory agents. The body transforms them into its own built-in anti-inflammatories, which can "turn off" the inflammatory reaction.

Neurological system health
Omega 3 is also vital for the health of the brain and nervous system. The cells have a special arrangement of fatty material on their outer surface called the myelin sheath, which is vital for sending and receiving messages. This can get damaged and needs adequate essential fatty acids for maintenance.

Research has also shown that omega 3 from oily fish can be beneficial in mental health and neurological system issues such as depression, memory enhancement, even behavior, and mood stability.

SARDINES

Heart & circulation
Sardines are another important member of the oily fish club. They have all the same omega-3 benefits as salmon.

SHRIMP

Skin health
Shrimp are incredibly rich in two vital minerals: zinc and selenium. Zinc helps regulate the oil-producing glands in the skin—if the skin is too oily or too dry, extra zinc can help balance things out a little. It is also vital for improved wound healing, as it regulates the activity of white blood cells involved in managing infection.

Selenium is also involved in wound healing and reduction of inflammation. Shrimp are also rich in a fat-soluble antioxidant called astaxanthin, which gives them their distinctive pink color. Astaxanthin accumulates in the fatty layer of the skin, where it can protect against premature aging and offer some anti-inflammatory activity. All of these things make shrimp a great choice for acne, eczema, and psoriasis.

Immune system health
The high zinc level in shrimp makes them a great food for the immune system. Zinc regulates many of the inner workings of white blood cells, the army of the immune system, ensuring they respond to the best of their ability to invaders or damaged cells and tissues.

TUNA

Heart & circulation
Several studies have found that tuna positively affects cholesterol levels. This is most likely due to the high omega-3 levels in fresh tuna. Canned tuna, although it's a great lean protein, is not a good source of omega 3, as all of the oils have been pressed out and sold to the nutritional supplements industry.

Skin health
Tuna is rich in the mineral selenium. This vital mineral is one of the key components in making the body's own antioxidant compounds. Selenium has proved beneficial for the health of the skin, and as an anti-inflammatory.

YOGURT

Digestive & immune system health
The live bacteria found in probiotic plain yogurt can help support the colony of good bacteria that naturally lives inside our digestive tract. This army of bacteria helps with almost every aspect of digestion. They also help regulate certain aspects of our immune response, too. Always choose good-quality, live probiotic plain yogurt.

GRAINS

BROWN RICE

Constipation
Like any fiber-rich food, brown rice will bulk out the stools, and therefore move more easily through the digestive tract.

Diabetes
Brown rice is a low-GI grain, which means it releases its energy very slowly. This helps keep blood sugar levels stable. Add a lean protein to the mix, and you have a very slow-release meal that is key to self-management of diabetes.

High cholesterol
It's mostly the fiber content that makes brown rice useful here. It helps move cholesterol out of the digestive tract, reducing the amount that gets absorbed into the bloodstream. There is a compound in brown rice known as gamma-oryzanol, which is also linked with lowering bad (LDL) cholesterol.

BULGUR WHEAT

Stress
Bulgur wheat is very rich in B vitamins. These vital nutrients are often deficient in Western diets, mainly because they are used rapidly during the stress response. They regulate many functions in the nervous system and adrenal glands. They are also vital for releasing energy from food, which is one reason why stress leaves us feeling depleted. B vitamins also seem to deliver a very calming effect. This is anecdotal, but quite commonly noticed.

High cholesterol & digestive system health
The fiber content of bulgur wheat makes it an ideal ingredient for digestive and heart health, as high-fiber foods will help remove cholesterol from the digestive tract before it can be absorbed.

CHICKPEAS

Reproductive system health
Chickpeas are packed with a group of compounds called isoflavones, which are very similar in chemical structure to estrogen, and so are a valuable dietary addition when dealing with issues such as problematic periods and menopause.

Skin health
Chickpeas, like all beans, are packed with the acne-fighting mineral zinc.

OATS

Heart & circulation
Oats contain a soluble fiber called beta-glucan. This has been clinically proven to lower cholesterol in the digestive tract. It does this by binding to cholesterol that has been released from the liver. Once

bound to it, it carries cholesterol out the body through the bowel before it has a chance to be absorbed into the bloodstream.

Constipation
The high fiber content of oats makes them an obvious choice for easing constipation. The fiber attracts water and begins to swell, which makes the bowel contents bigger and bulkier. This helps stimulate the stretch receptors in the gut wall, which causes it to contract in a process known as peristalsis, helping to move bowel contents along more effectively.

Stress
Oats are very rich in B vitamins, which are essential for supporting the body during stressful times. They support adrenal gland function and nervous system activity, and are essential for energy production at a cellular level. They are rapidly depleted during stressful times, which can leave us feeling washed out very quickly.

QUINOA

Diabetes & blood sugar stability
Quinoa, a grain that originates in South America, is a complete protein, and contains all the essential amino acids we need to make our own proteins. Unlike many grains, quinoa is low in carbohydrates and is very low GI. This means it will release its energy slowly, and won't cause blood sugar spikes, making it a perfect alternative to rice for anyone who wants to stabilize their blood sugar levels more effectively.

RED LENTILS

High cholesterol
Red lentils contain a high percentage of soluble fiber. This is not only helpful for digestion, but also helps remove cholesterol from the gut, and thereby reduces the amount that gets absorbed into the bloodstream through the digestive tract.

Constipation
The high fiber content also helps keep things moving through the digestive tract properly.

NUTS & SEEDS

BRAZIL NUTS

Allergies & inflammation
Brazil nuts are sometimes deemed unhealthy because of their oil content. But that's a big mistake—they are very rich in the mineral selenium, which plays many roles in the body, including regulating the inflammatory response and some aspects of the allergic response. Selenium increases the production of some of the body's own built-in antioxidants.

COCONUT

Colds & flu
Coconut oil has put people off a bit in recent years because of its high saturated fat content. But this is unjustified in my view, as these fats can be very beneficial. It's actually one of the best choices of cooking fats, and the fats won't break down into trans fats at high temperatures. One of the main fats found in coconut oil is a substance called lauric acid, which has been shown to have some interesting antiviral properties. It actually blocks the way viruses enter our cells and multiply.

FLAX SEEDS

Anti-inflammatory
Thanks to the very high levels of omega-3 fatty acids, flax seeds (also known as linseeds) can deliver some impressive anti-inflammatory activity. This is because they help to increase the production of the body's own anti-inflammatory compounds, and inhibit the production of pro-inflammatory compounds.

PUMPKIN SEEDS

High cholesterol
Pumpkin seeds are very rich in a compound called beta-sitosterol, which is added to those cholesterol-lowering drinks we see advertised so often. It works by blocking the absorption of cholesterol through the gut, and has had vast amounts of clinical research conducted on it.

Fungal conditions
Pumpkin seeds contain curcubitin, which has shown some interesting antifungal activity. It is believed to be useful for digestive parasites such as candida. Although I'm sceptical about the amount of attention paid to candida by the natural health world, it can be a problem, and this compound may well be a good option.

Acne
Pumpkin seeds are very high in zinc, which helps regulate the sebaceous glands. This can help even out oily acne-prone skin.

WALNUTS

Heart & circulation
Walnuts are great for heart health for two reasons. Firstly, they are rich in vitamin E, which is a natural blood thinner. Eating foods rich in vitamin E may be protective against strokes and heart attacks. They are also rich in omega 3, which has a further blood thinning action, and also helps to improve the balance between bad (LDL) and good (HDL) cholesterol.

BASICS & FLAVORINGS

ANISE

Bloating
Anise candies have traditionally been used to settle the digestion. The essential oil anethol, which creates the familiar aroma, can work as a muscle relaxant, helping to relax the walls of the digestive tract and regulate bowel movements. Herbalists describe anise oil as carminative, which means it can help to disperse gas.

Coughs
Anethol is also believed to be a bronchiodilator, which means that it opens up the airways in the lungs. This can offer some relief for dry, irritated coughs.

BASIL

Digestive system health
Basil has quite complex chemistry, and the volatile oils that provide its distinctive flavor relax the muscular walls of the small intestines, and can therefore ease digestive cramps and bloating.

CACAO

The word cocoa is actually a bastardization of the word *cacao*, which is the botanical name for the bean from which chocolate is made. This potent food is, believe it or not, one of the most nutrient-rich foods on the planet. Raw cacao powder is a very different animal from your standard grocery store cocoa powder. In its raw and unprocessed state, it has over 1,500 beneficial compounds in it. Once processed (for example, into ordinary unsweetened cocoa), only five remain, the main one being caffeine!

Heart & circulation
Cacao is packed with a group of compounds called flavonoids. These compounds have been very widely researched and are known to cause the cells that line our blood vessels to release high levels of a compound called nitric oxide, which causes the muscles in the blood vessel walls to relax. When they relax, the blood vessel widens, which lowers the pressure within it. Cacao is very high in the mineral magnesium, which also encourages relaxation of the smooth muscle in vessel walls.

Mental health & neurological system
Raw cacao is very rich in two powerful compounds that have an interesting effect on the mind and mood. The first is called anandamide, and is also naturally produced in our brain. It enhances motivation and pleasure, and is said to give feelings of bliss.

The next, phenylethylamine (PEA for short), is a powerful mood elevator. It is also present in ordinary chocolate, but in much lower concentrations than in raw cacao. It is quite rapidly broken down by an enzyme before it gets chance to reach the brain. However, the high concentration of PEA in raw cacao does allow a small amount to get through and have neurological effects, albeit mild.

Natural energy boost
Cacao contains a stimulant compound called theobromine, a close cousin of caffeine. It is a stimulant, but it seems to have less of a "burn out" aftereffect than caffeine. I would still avoid overconsumption, though.

CARDAMOM

Bloating & wind
Like many aromatic spices, cardamom can be a godsend if you are feeling bloated and gassy. The essential oils that create its divine, aromatic flavor help reduce gas and regulate peristalsis, the natural rhythmic contractions of the gut. This can offer relief of symptoms of digestive difficulty by ensuring that everything is moving along as it should be.

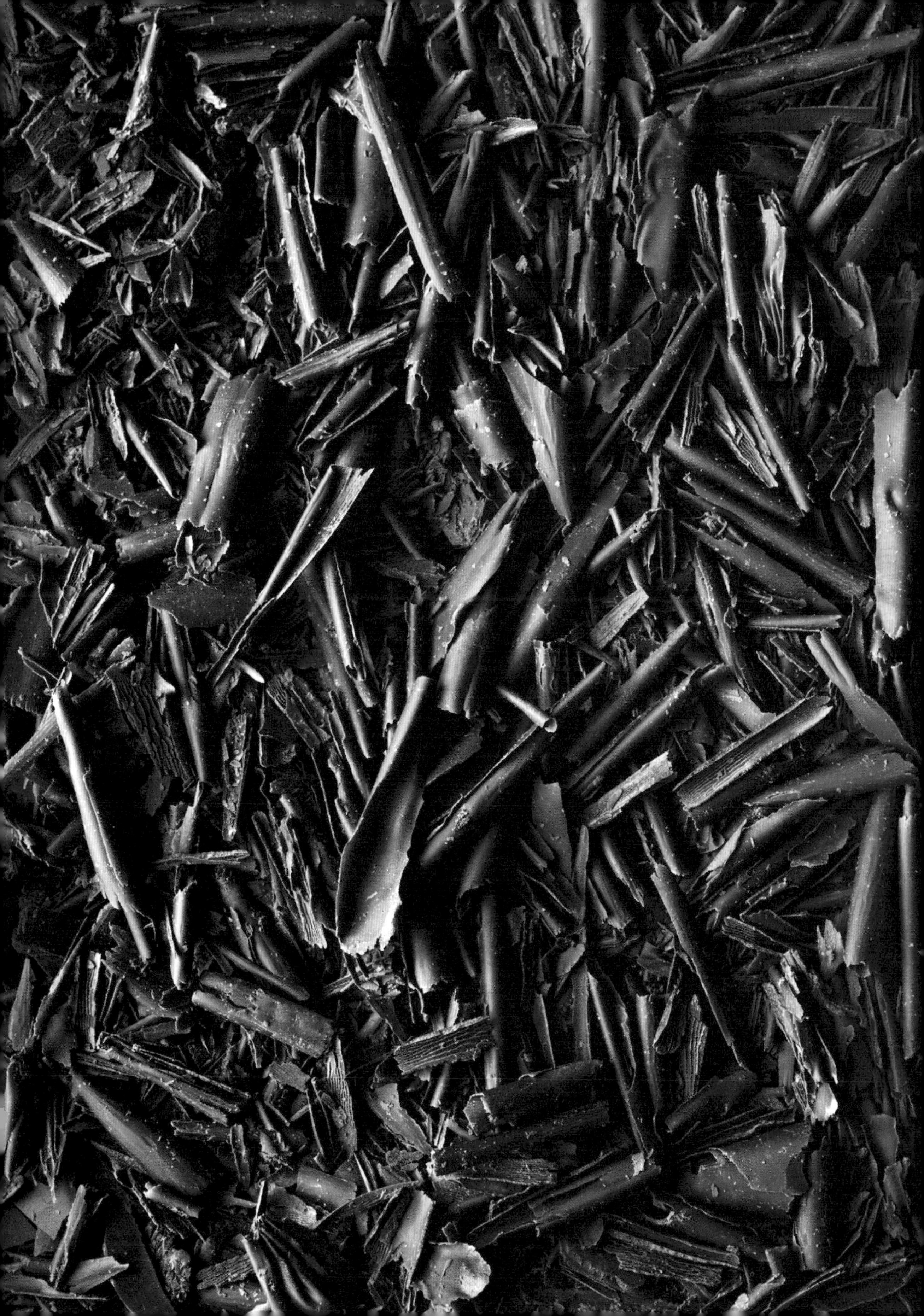

CHILI PEPPERS

High blood pressure & circulation
Chili peppers contain a powerful phytochemical called capsaicin, which gives them their intense heat. Capsaicin causes the cells that line the inside of our blood vessels to secrete a chemical called nitric oxide, which is naturally produced by these cells (chili peppers just give them a kick in the right direction). Nitric oxide then tells the muscles in the blood vessel walls to relax, so the vessel gets wider.

This has two benefits: firstly, the wider the blood vessel, the lower the pressure within it, and secondly, circulation to the extremities is improved.

Pain reduction
The capsaicin in chili peppers also has painkilling effects. Firstly, the heat from the peppers stimulates the release of our own natural endorphins, which can lower our perception of pain to a degree. Secondly, it can reduce the levels of something called substance P, a chemical released by nerves that carries pain signals.

CINNAMON

Metabolic system health & blood sugar levels
Some evidence has come to light in recent years that suggests that cinnamon may play a role in blood-sugar balance, which might help with many conditions. It's thought that compounds in cinnamon can actually make cells slightly more receptive to insulin, the hormone that tells them to take up sugar to use as energy.

CORIANDER

Digestive system health
Coriander is frequently used as a carminative, which means that it can help with several digestive conditions, from bloating and gas to nausea.

GARLIC

Heart & circulation
Garlic contains some seriously potent chemical activity. It contains a powerful compound called ajoene, which interacts with something called the platelet aggregation factor, a compound in the body that regulates the rate and extent to which blood clots. Some surgeons and dentists even advise patients against eating garlic a couple of days prior to surgery in case it increases their bleeding. On a day-to-day basis, however, it can offer protection against clotting, helpful against strokes and heart attacks.

Colds & flu
Garlic contains a group of powerful essential oils—these are what make you smell like Buffy the Vampire Slayer's inside pocket when you've eaten too much of it. These oils can only be removed from the body through the breath, rather than the usual routes of elimination through the bowels, and urine. As we breathe out they move through the respiratory tract and can kill off bugs and viruses, such as those that can cause colds and flu.

Anti-inflammatory
Raw garlic is actually a reasonably effective anti-inflammatory, due to a compound called diallyl sulfide. This compound breaks down drastically during cooking, though.

GINGER

Anti-inflammatory
One of the true kings of the food realm, ginger is one of the most powerful anti-inflammatories there is. The strong, spicy essential oils that give it its spicy flavor have been shown by many studies to interrupt certain aspects of the chemical reaction that occurs when inflammation is triggered.

Nausea
Ginger has a longstanding reputation as a useful remedy for the treatment of mild nausea, from morning sickness to motion sickness. It isn't clear how it does this, but many people believe it works by stimulating the production of digestive juices.

HONEY

Honey is a better choice of sweetener than processed sugar (in other words, the granulated stuff you put in your tea), as it releases its energy slightly more slowly, and also contains a fair amount of nutrition along with its calories. That said, I'm still a strong advocate for reducing sugar consumption, natural or otherwise. Honey delivers antioxidant and anti-inflammatory properties, some varieties more than others.

Immune system health
Honey is recognized as a bacteriostatic compound, meaning that it halts bacterial growth. When applied topically (on the surface), the dense concentration of sugar in honey creates an environment that stops the replication and activity of bacteria. This is why honey plasters are still used in hospitals to reduce infection in pressure sores and venous ulcers. Honey also contains an array of compounds such as resins, polyphenols, caffeic acids, and so on, which all deliver a degree of antiviral and immuno-supportive activities.

HORSERADISH

Asthma & coughs
Horseradish is believed to be a bronchodilator, meaning that it helps to open up the airways, which may go some way toward relieving mild asthma symptoms (absolutely never in place of medication, though), as well as chesty coughs.

Respiratory infections
The spicy compounds in horseradish also work as a mild irritant to the upper respiratory tract, causing the mucous membranes to secrete a thinner mucous, which helps to dislodge the thicker mucous that can arise due to infection.

LEMONGRASS

High blood pressure & circulation
The oils in lemon grass that give it its distinctive flavor are believed to relax the muscular walls of blood vessels. This makes the vessels a bit wider and enhances circulation to the extremities.

MINT

Bloating & gas
The essential oils in mint, such as menthol, help relax the wall of the digestive tract, and also to break down and disperse gas. If I ever feel a little bloated, I turn to mint every time; it really is a very rapid remedy indeed.

OLIVE OIL

Heart & circulation
Olive oil has been touted as a healthy oil for centuries, and in many cultures. Modern research has confirmed some rather beneficial properties in this widely used oil. Olive oil is very high in an omega-9 fatty acid called oleic acid, which has been shown in a lot of research to lower total (LDL) cholesterol levels, and improve the ratio between good (LDL) and bad (HDL) cholesterol. It also contains some unique antioxidants called polyphenols, which help to reduce platelet aggregation (basically, reducing clotting).

Asthma, arthritis & eczema
I always recommend that anyone with inflammatory conditions should only use olive oil in their cooking. Excessive consumption of omega-6 fatty acids is a big issue in the Western world, particularly in the vegetable oils that are now so widely used. In our quest to reduce saturated fat levels, many of us are consuming more unsaturated vegetable oils, most of which are almost pure omega 6.

Now, omega 6 is a vital fatty acid, but if we consume too much (and most of us do), it can trigger low-grade inflammation in tissues, which can cause long-term damage. It can also worsen inflammatory conditions, such as arthritis. Reducing omega 6, along with increased intake of omega 3, can have a powerful effect upon inflammatory conditions, and getting a balance between the two is vital. Olive oil contains mostly omega-9 fatty acids, so using it in food helps us to control the amount of omega 6 we consume.

PARSLEY

Kidney & urinary system health
As well as being very high in vitamin C, parsley can be useful in conditions such as fluid retention, urinary tract infections like cystitis, and even for giving the kidneys a bit of support after a night on the tiles. It contains a very potent essential oil that works as a mild irritant for the nephron (the kidney's filtration system), and increases the rate of fluid movement across this filter, thereby increasing urinary output.

PEPPERCORNS

Digestive system health
Black pepper is believed to be a good remedy for constipation,

as it can act as a mild stimulant of peristalsis, the rhythmical contractions in the gut that keep everything moving. In Ayurvedic medicine, pepper is also used to stimulate appetite.

ROSEMARY

Anti-inflammatory
Rosemary contains a very powerful anti-inflammatory compound (albeit in small amounts), called rosmarinic acid, which blocks certain compounds that stimulate the inflammatory response.

High blood pressure & circulation
The essential oils in rosemary are thought to be vasodilatory, which means that they help widen the blood vessels. As the vessel widens, the pressure within it is reduced.

Another benefit is that it will enhance circulation to the extremities. This is why some traditional medical practices use rosemary for treating cold fingers and toes, Raynaud's disease, and even to enhance memory (although the jury's still out on that one).

SAGE

Bloating & gas
The oils in sage, which give it its pungent flavor, are very powerful carminatives. This means that they help dispel gas and bloating, helping to relieve digestive discomfort.

THYME

Neurological system health
A compound in thyme has been shown to increase the amount of DHA, a vital essential fatty acid, in nervous tissue. This fat is a vital structural component of these tissues, and low levels can be detrimental to the normal functioning of each nerve cell.

Bacterial infections
Thyme has always been my first port of call for upper respiratory tract infections. The complex chemistry that gives thyme its powerful flavor and aroma, including the essential oil thymol, has been identified as having potent antibacterial activity, hence the traditional usage for conditions such as throat infections.

TURMERIC

Anti-inflammatory
Turmeric is one of the kings of medicinal food. The chemicals that provide its vivid, bright-orange color are a group of compounds called curcuminoids. These have been studied for decades and are known to reduce inflammation by blocking an enzyme involved in triggering inflammation. Turmeric is very powerful indeed, and some studies have even compared the effectiveness of extracts of turmeric with some pharmaceutical drugs.

Liver health
The curcuminoids in turmeric have also been shown to help protect the liver. Studies have shown that they can reduce inflammation and damage to hepatocytes, the liver cells, caused by chemical irritants such as alcohol and pollutants.

Heart & circulation
Compounds in turmeric are also believed to have a degree of anticoagulant activity. This means they can regulate the rate and extent to which blood clots, which may offer some degree of protection against heart attack and stroke.

RECIPES

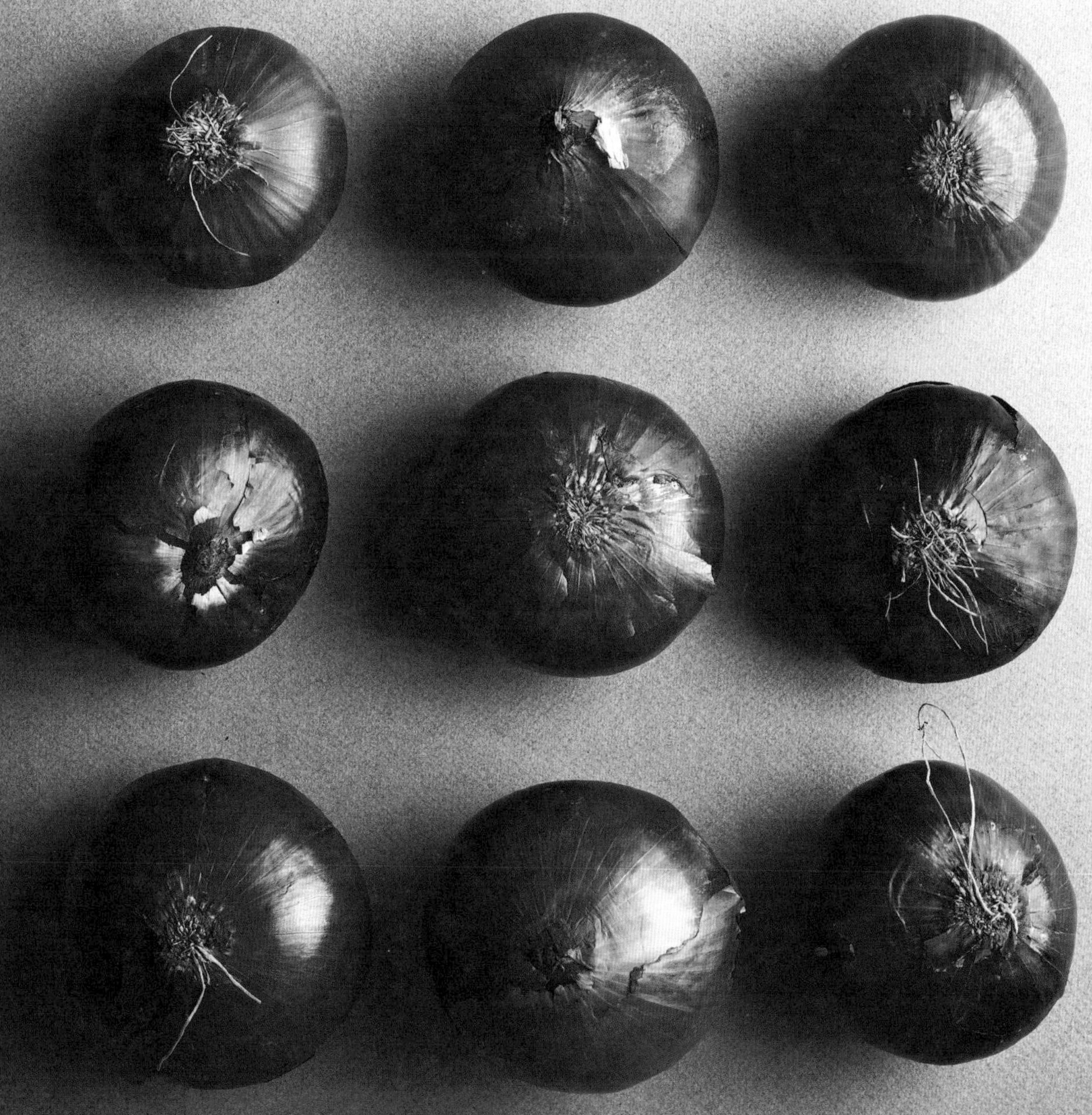

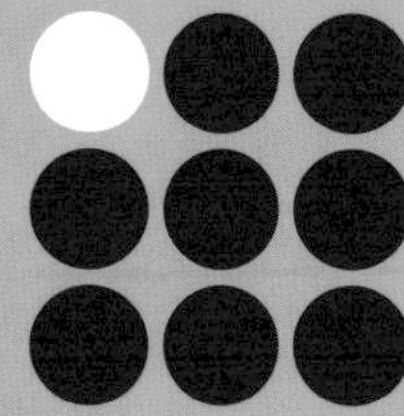

Breakfast & brunch

It's true what they say: breakfast really is the most important meal of the day. Breakfast is also when we're most likely to consume utter trash, so it's vital to ensure that you're prepared, and have plenty of good-quality options available.

Now, you may find that you're not very hungry first thing in the morning, and it might take a while to get your appetite kick-started. However, it's still a good idea to have a small piece of fruit in the early morning, just to top off blood sugar and wake the metabolism from its slumber. These dishes are perfect first thing, or are equally well placed as midmorning fare, too. They are all easily doubled to serve 2 or 4.

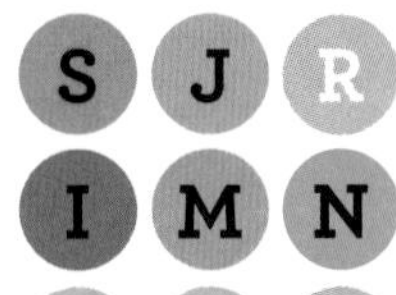

SKIN
JOINTS & BONES *Osteoporosis, Rickets*
IMMUNE SYSTEM
METABOLIC SYSTEM *Diabetes (Type 2)*
MENTAL HEALTH & NERVOUS SYSTEM *Anxiety*

Spinach and feta scramble

This makes for a gorgeous start to the day, and contains three of my favorite ingredients in one hit. It's dense in nutrients and guaranteed to keep you going until lunchtime.

SERVES 1

½ tablespoon olive oil
2 handfuls baby spinach
2 large free-range eggs
½ cup feta cheese, crumbled
small bunch fresh chives, minced
sea salt and black pepper

Heat the olive oil in a pan over medium heat, add the spinach, and cook for 3 to 4 minutes, or until wilted.

Crack the eggs into a bowl, season with salt and pepper, and whisk them together. Pour them into the pan with the spinach and add the crumbled feta. Stir gently over medium-low heat until the eggs have scrambled. Sprinkle with the chopped chives and serve immediately.

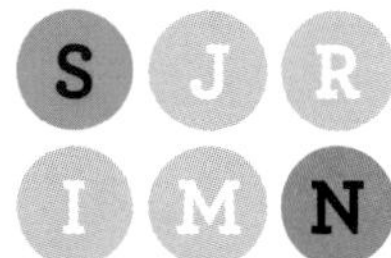

SKIN *Acne*
MENTAL HEALTH & NERVOUS SYSTEM *Stress*
HEART & CIRCULATION *High cholesterol*
DIGESTIVE SYSTEM *Constipation*

Blast-off breakfast bars

These bars are a great solution when you just need to grab something and get out the door, or if you don't feel ready for anything heavy early in the morning. They're low GI and packed with complex carbohydrates, protein, and vital "good" fats. Guaranteed to launch you into your day! Goji berries are available in most health food stores.

MAKES 6 TO 8 BARS

light olive oil, for greasing
2 tablespoons honey, plus extra for drizzling
4 tablespoons coconut oil
3 tablespoons peanut butter (a good-quality one, with no added salt or sugar)
2 cups rolled oats
3 tablespoons ground flax seeds
1 tablespoon pumpkin seeds
1 tablespoon goji berries
2 tablespoons chopped dates
1 tablespoon chopped dried figs

Preheat the oven to 350°F and lightly grease a 9-inch square baking pan.

Melt the honey, coconut oil, and peanut butter together over gentle heat in a pan. Remove from the heat, add the rest of the ingredients (setting a few seeds and dates aside to sprinkle over the top), and stir well to form a sticky mixture. Press the mixture firmly into the prepared pan. Sprinkle with reserved pumpkin seeds and dates.

Bake in the oven for 10 to 15 minutes, or until golden brown. Let cool completely before cutting into bars. Store in an airtight container. They will keep for up to a week. Serve with a little honey drizzled over, if you like.

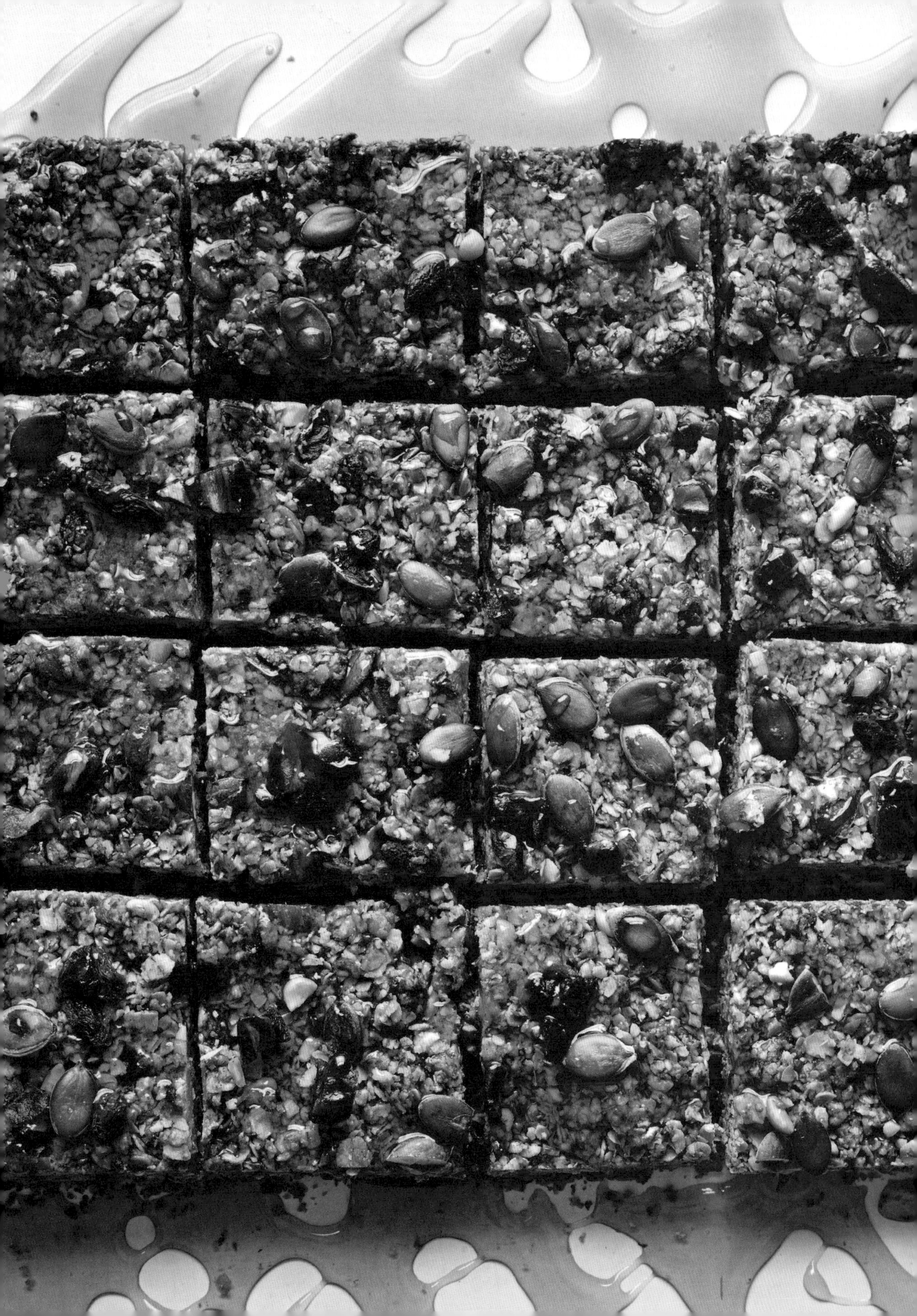

S J R
I M N
H D U

HEART & CIRCULATION *High cholesterol*
DIGESTIVE SYSTEM *Hemorrhoids*

Probiotic layer crunch

This is a nice, simple breakfast that checks all the right boxes to start your day off well: complex carbohydrates, vitamins, and minerals, low GI . . . and it looks rather nice too! The quantities are variable depending on the size of the serving glass you're using. You can make it as big or as small as you like.

SERVES 1 TO 100

fresh berries (blueberries, chopped strawberries, blackberries, or whatever floats your boat)
rolled oats
pumpkin seeds
live probiotic plain yogurt
ground cinnamon, for sprinkling (optional)
honey, for drizzling (optional)

Find a nice-sized glass—a large tumbler, for example.

Begin with a thin layer of fresh berries. Top this with a thin layer of rolled oats, then a thin layer of pumpkin seeds, then finally a layer of yogurt. Repeat this process as many times as is necessary to fill your vessel of choice. You can add a little pinch of cinnamon and a drizzle of honey at the end to jazz things up a bit.

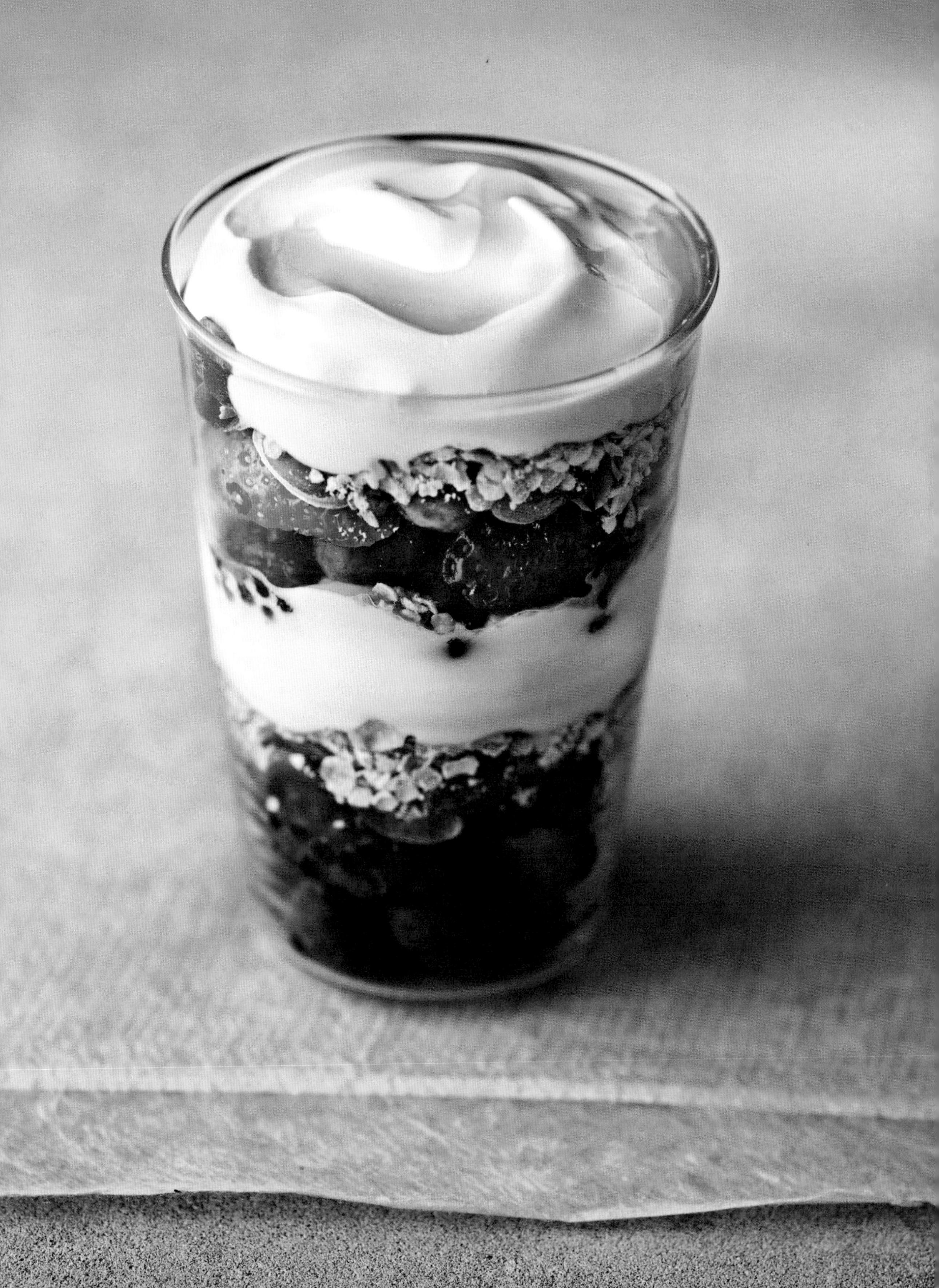

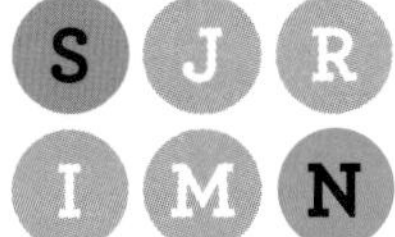

SKIN
MENTAL HEALTH & NERVOUS SYSTEM *Depression*
DIGESTIVE SYSTEM *Bloating*
REPRODUCTIVE & URINARY SYSTEMS *Polycystic ovary syndrome*

Herbed Mediterranean frittata

This is a great dish for those mornings when you wake up and feel so ravenous that you could eat anything in sight. It's big on flavor, big on nutrition.

SERVES 1 TO 2

olive oil, for cooking
6 cherry tomatoes
¼ red onion, finely sliced
1 garlic clove, minced
5–6 black olives, pitted
3 large free-range eggs
sea salt and black pepper
small handful fresh parsley, minced
small handful fresh basil, minced
small handful fresh mint, minced

Preheat the broiler. Heat a dash of olive oil in a skillet or omelet pan over medium heat. Add the cherry tomatoes, onion, and garlic to the skillet, season with salt, and cook until the onion has softened. At this stage, throw in the olives.

Whisk the eggs in a small bowl, season with salt and pepper, and stir in the chopped herbs. Pour the eggs into the skillet.

Keep the skillet on a consistent medium-high heat for 3 to 4 minutes, enough time to cook the lower portion of the frittata. At this point, place the pan underneath the preheated broiler to cook the top part of the frittata. To check if it's cooked, insert a knife in it. If you can see a lot of runny egg, cook it for a minute or two longer. Let stand for a minute before serving.

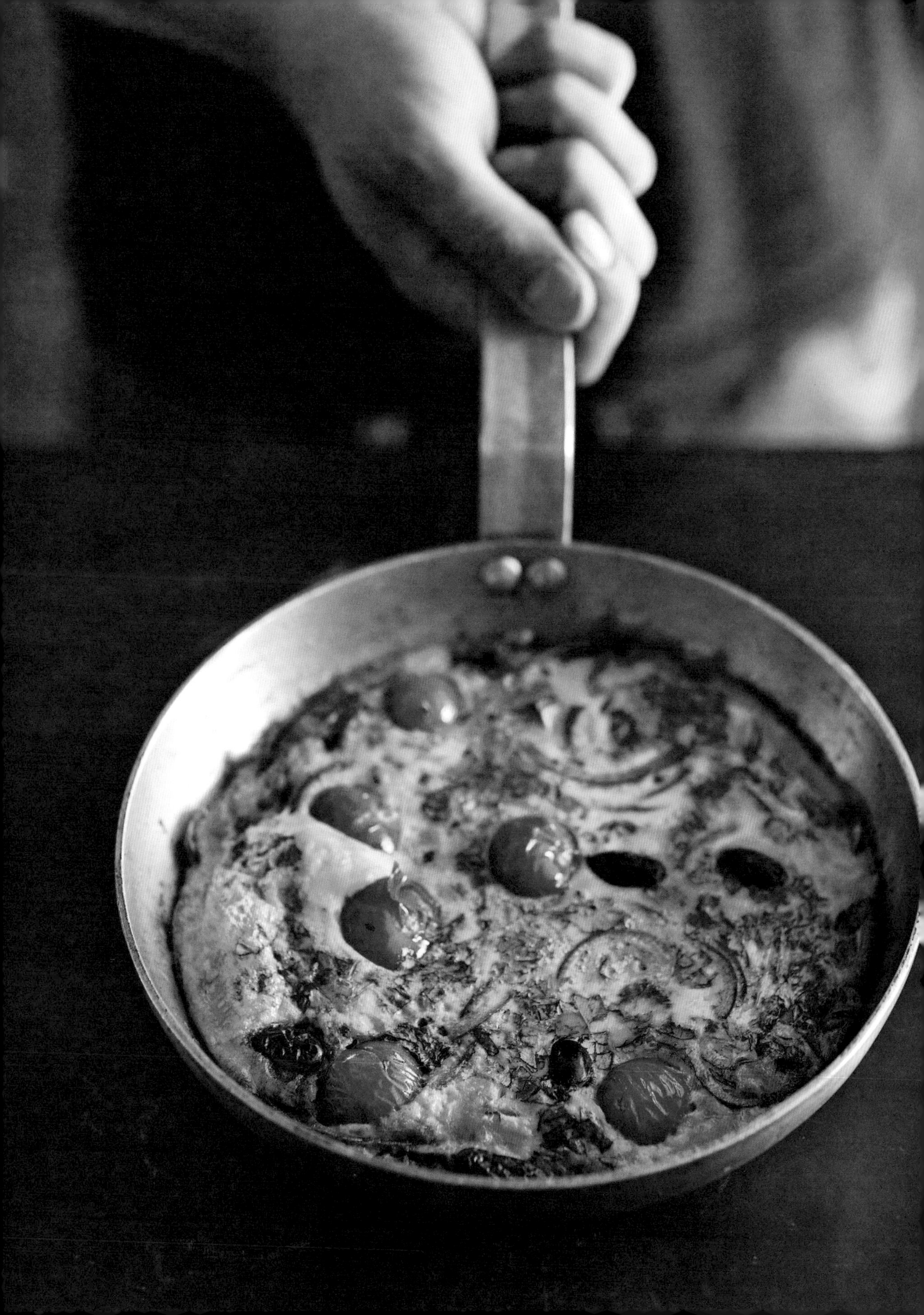

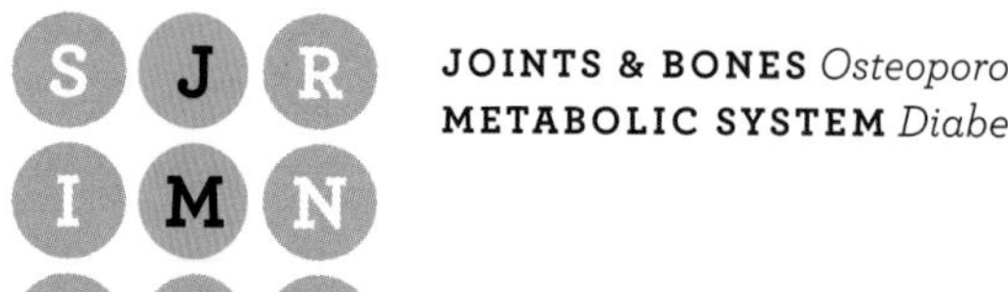

JOINTS & BONES *Osteoporosis, Rickets*
METABOLIC SYSTEM *Diabetes (Type 2)*

Easy eggs florentine

This is a simple but tasty breakfast or brunch. It's fresh, vibrant, and surprisingly filling. Leave out the hollandaise sauce if you want to be virtuous—but we all deserve the occasional weekend treat! Easily doubled for two.

SERVES 1

olive oil, for cooking
large handful baby spinach leaves
sea salt and black pepper
1 teaspoon wine vinegar
3 large free-range eggs
6 tablespoons butter
juice of ¼ lemon
1 sprig fresh dill, chopped
2 slices rye or whole grain bread

Heat a little olive oil in a pan over medium heat, add the spinach, and cook for 3 to 4 minutes, or until wilted. Season with salt and pepper.

Bring a small pan of water to a simmer, turn down the heat so that the water is barely bubbling, and add the vinegar. Crack 2 eggs, one at a time, into a cup and then slide them gently into the water. Poach for 3 to 4 minutes.

Meanwhile, make the hollandaise sauce by melting the butter gently in a small pan. Place an egg yolk and the lemon juice in a small food processor or blender and process until smooth. Add the hot melted butter, still processing, to make a thick sauce. Season with salt and pepper and stir in some of the chopped dill.

Toast the bread and drain the spinach in a strainer. Stir in the remaining fresh dill and place the spinach on top of the toast. Remove the eggs from the water with a slotted spoon and place on top of the spinach. Top with the hollandaise sauce, season, and serve immediately.

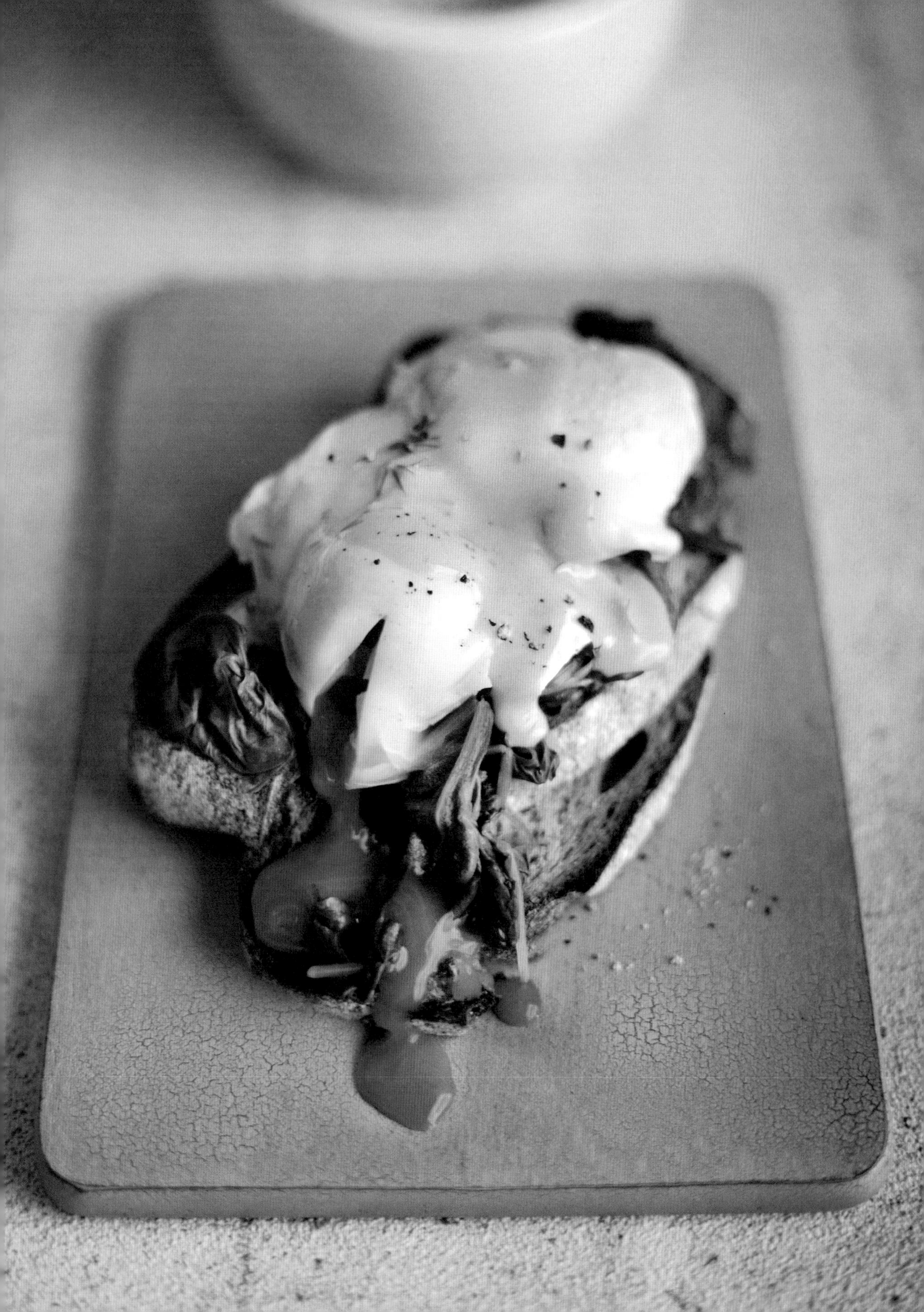

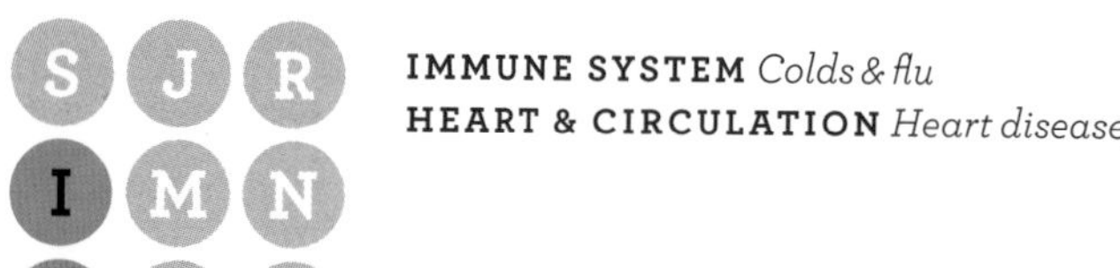

Spinach, tomato, and shiitake mushrooms on toast

This is great when you crave something really tasty but can't be bothered to slave away in the kitchen for ages.

SERVES 1

olive oil, for cooking
1 large garlic clove, minced
6–7 shiitake mushrooms, sliced
4–5 cherry tomatoes, halved
handful baby spinach
1 slice whole grain bread
sea salt and black pepper

Heat a little olive oil over medium heat in a large pan, add the garlic, and cook gently for a minute or so, until softened.

Add the shiitake mushrooms and cook, stirring, for 2 minutes, then add the tomatoes and season with salt and pepper. Cook for 4 to 5 minutes, or until the mushrooms have softened. Add the spinach and cook for a minute or two longer, until it has wilted.

Meanwhile, toast the bread. Top with the mushroom mixture and serve immediately.

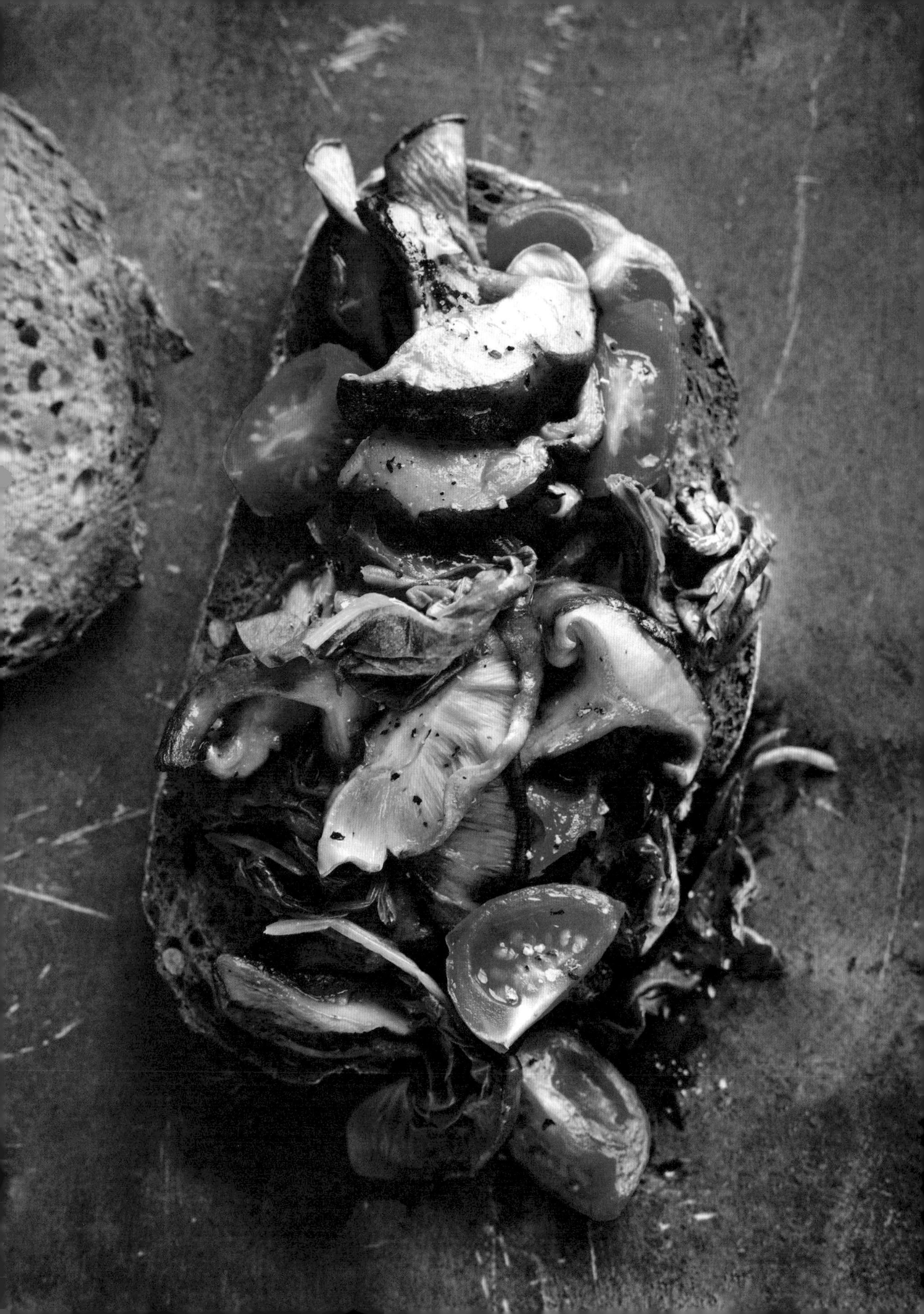

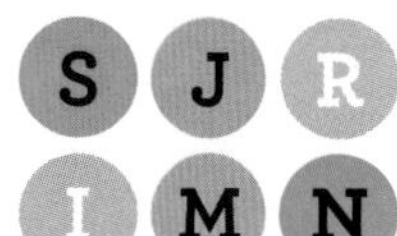

SKIN *Acne*
JOINTS & BONES *Arthritis*
METABOLIC SYSTEM *Diabetes (Type 2)*
MENTAL HEALTH & NERVOUS SYSTEM *Migraine*
HEART & CIRCULATION *High blood pressure, High cholesterol*
DIGESTIVE SYSTEM *Crohn's disease*

Asparagus and smoked salmon egg dippers

There's something a little bit posh and decadent about this dish, and it's great for so many body systems. It makes a lovely appetizer, or even a between-meal snack.

SERVES 1

6 asparagus spears, trimmed
1 large free-range egg
2 ounces smoked salmon

Bring a small pan of water to a boil, then lower the heat to a gentle, rolling boil. Drop the asparagus into the water for 4 to 5 minutes, just long enough for it to turn a bright, vivid green. Remove, drain, and dry on paper towels.

Place the egg in the boiling water and boil for 6 minutes, for a soft-boiled egg (hard white, soft yolk).

While the egg is cooking, cut the smoked salmon into strips, and wrap them around the middle of the asparagus spears.

Remove the egg from the water and place it in an egg cup. Remove the top to expose the runny yolk, ready for dipping. For a hard-boiled egg with a fully set yolk, cook for 10 minutes.

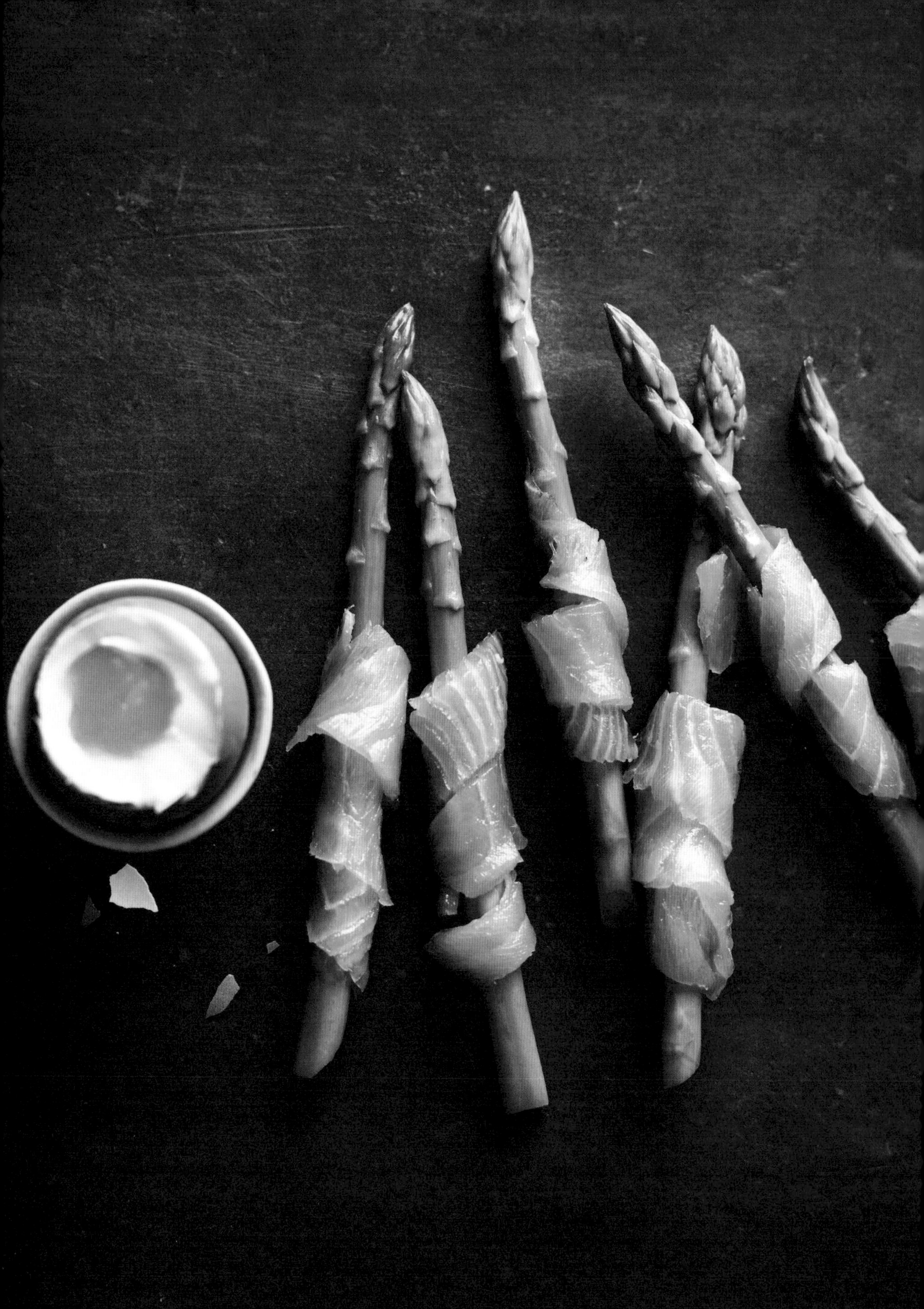

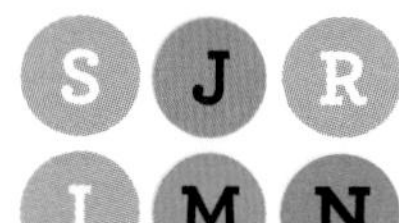
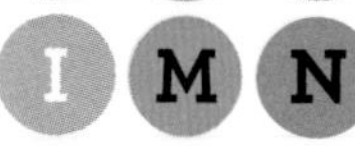
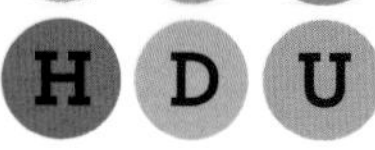

JOINTS & BONES *Arthritis, Bursitis*
METABOLIC SYSTEM *Diabetes (Type 2)*
MENTAL HEALTH & NERVOUS SYSTEM *Depression*
HEART & CIRCULATION *Heart disease, High cholesterol*
DIGESTIVE SYSTEM *Hemorrhoids*
REPRODUCTIVE & URINARY SYSTEMS *Menopause, Polycystic ovary syndrome*

Kick-starter kedgeree

I first tasted kedgeree as a youngster and just loved it then and there. It's very filling and packed with nutrients. Guaranteed to keep you going for hours on end!

SERVES 1

olive oil, for cooking
½ small red onion, minced
½ red bell pepper, chopped
1 teaspoon curry powder
½ teaspoon turmeric
1 red chili pepper, thinly sliced
generous ⅓ cup brown basmati rice
sea salt and black pepper
1 large free-range egg
handful baby spinach
1 smoked mackerel fillet (about 5 ounces), broken into small pieces
1 tablespoon live probiotic plain yogurt

Heat a little olive oil over medium heat in a large pan, add the onion and red pepper, and cook gently until softened, about 5 minutes.

Add the curry powder, turmeric, chili pepper, and rice and stir for a few minutes to toast the spices slightly. Add enough water to cover the rice, season with salt and pepper, and simmer, covered, over medium-high heat for about 20 minutes, or until the rice has softened. You may need to top off the water now and then during the cooking time.

Meanwhile, cover the egg with water in a small pan, bring to a boil, and boil for 7 minutes. Drain under cold water and let cool before peeling and cutting into quarters lengthwise.

Just before the rice is cooked, stir in the baby spinach and cook for a couple more minutes to wilt the spinach. When the rice is cooked, stir in the flaked mackerel and yogurt. Serve with the egg wedges on top.

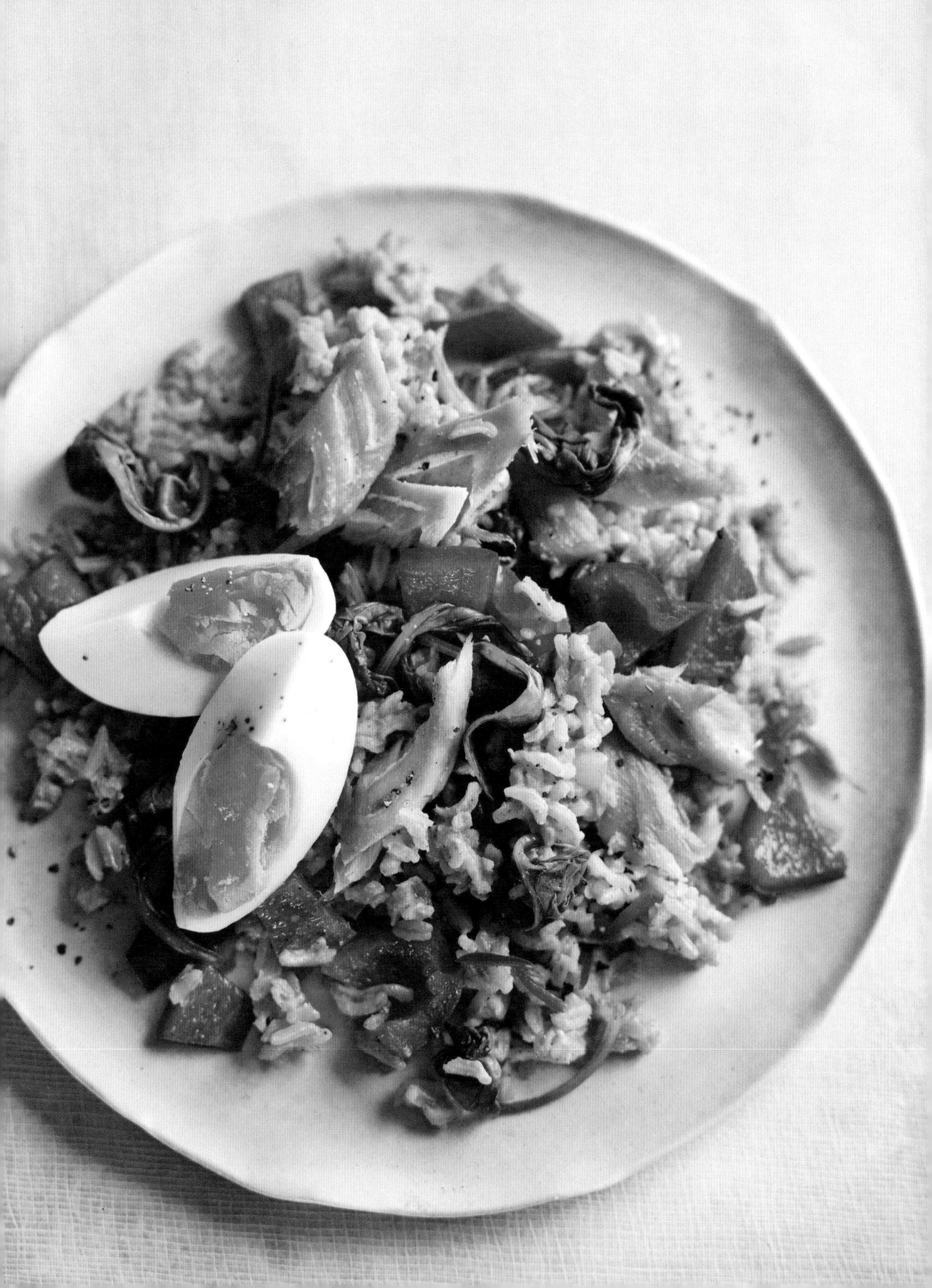

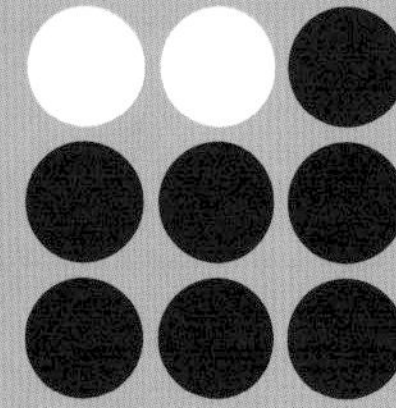

Soups

Soup is one of the best, most warming comfort foods there is, and one of the most effective ways of getting lots of good ingredients into your diet. Fresh herbs and spices, vegetables and aromatics such as garlic are all soup staples and nutritional powerhouses, enabling you to create a dish that provides masses of health benefits in a very small portion size. Soups freeze very well and are easy to transport, so they're ideal for taking to work or on long journeys to make sure you have some ultra-nutritional food on hand.

If you feel a bit full and bloated after eating these soups, it's a temporary effect and means the good bacteria in your gut are starting to have a party. Their numbers are increasing and the colony is getting stronger. Both of them are wonderful for the digestion.

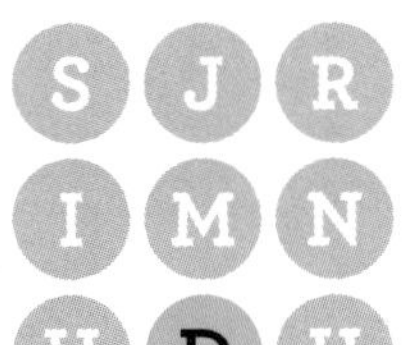

DIGESTIVE SYSTEM
Constipation, Bloating

The digestive dynamo

SERVES 3 TO 4

olive oil, for cooking
1 large white onion, minced
2 garlic cloves, minced
10½ ounces Jerusalem artichokes, roughly diced, skin left on
2 parsnips, roughly diced, skin left on
about 2 cups vegetable stock (made with stock cubes or bouillon powder)
sea salt and black pepper
3–4 tablespoons live probiotic plain yogurt

Heat a little olive oil in a large pan, add the onion and garlic, and cook over medium-high heat for 4 to 5 minutes, or until the onion is soft and translucent.

Add the Jerusalem artichokes and parsnips and enough vegetable stock to cover them. Simmer for about 15 minutes, or until the parsnips and artichokes are tender.

Season with salt and pepper. Transfer in batches to a blender and process into a smooth, velvety soup. Serve with a dollop of yogurt and some freshly ground black pepper.

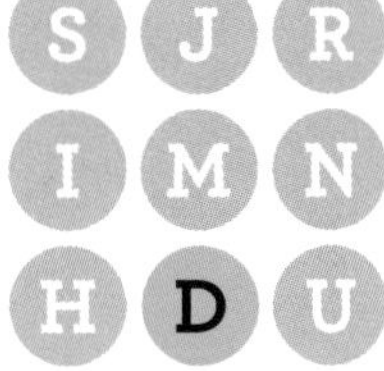

DIGESTIVE SYSTEM
Bloating

Fennel and celery root soup

SERVES 3 TO 4

olive oil, for cooking
1 large white onion, minced
1 garlic clove, minced
2 large fennel bulbs, coarsely chopped
½ large celery root, roughly diced, skin left on
1 potato, diced, skin left on
generous 2 cups vegetable stock (made with stock cubes or bouillon powder)
sea salt and black pepper
1 teaspoon fennel seeds (optional)

Heat a little olive oil in a large pan, add the onion and garlic, and cook over medium-high heat for 4 to 5 minutes, or until the onion has softened.

Add the fennel, celery root, and potato, and add enough vegetable stock to cover. Simmer until the potato and celery root feel soft, about 10 minutes.

Season with salt and pepper. Transfer in batches to a blender and process into a velvety smooth soup. Sprinkle with fennel seeds, if using.

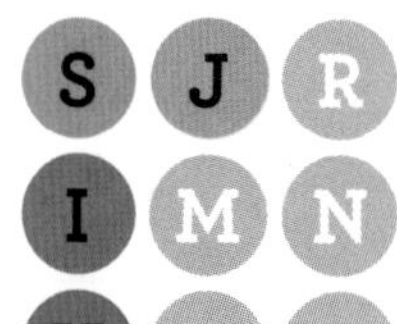

SKIN *Acne*
JOINTS & BONES *Arthritis*
IMMUNE SYSTEM *Colds & flu*
HEART & CIRCULATION *High cholesterol*

The famous flu fighter

This one-pot wonder of a soup is an absolute powerhouse when it comes to dealing with colds and flu. Don't be put off by the goji berries—these sweet treats were once hard to find, and cost a fortune, but thankfully they can now be found in any health food store at a reasonable price.

SERVES 4

1 red onion, minced
1 green chili pepper, minced
4 garlic cloves, minced
2-inch piece fresh ginger, minced
2 tablespoons olive oil
2 medium sweet potatoes, diced, skins left on
4 ounces shiitake mushrooms, sliced
2 handfuls goji berries
vegetable stock, to cover
salt and black pepper

Put the onion, chili pepper, garlic, and ginger in a large pan with the olive oil. Cook over medium-high heat for about 5 minutes, until the onion softens.

Add the sweet potatoes and mushrooms to the pan along with the goji berries. Stir well, then add enough vegetable stock to cover all the ingredients. Simmer well for 10 to 15 minutes, until the potato is soft. Season with salt and pepper.

Carefully add the soup to a blender in batches, and blend into a smooth, vivid orange, spicy soup.

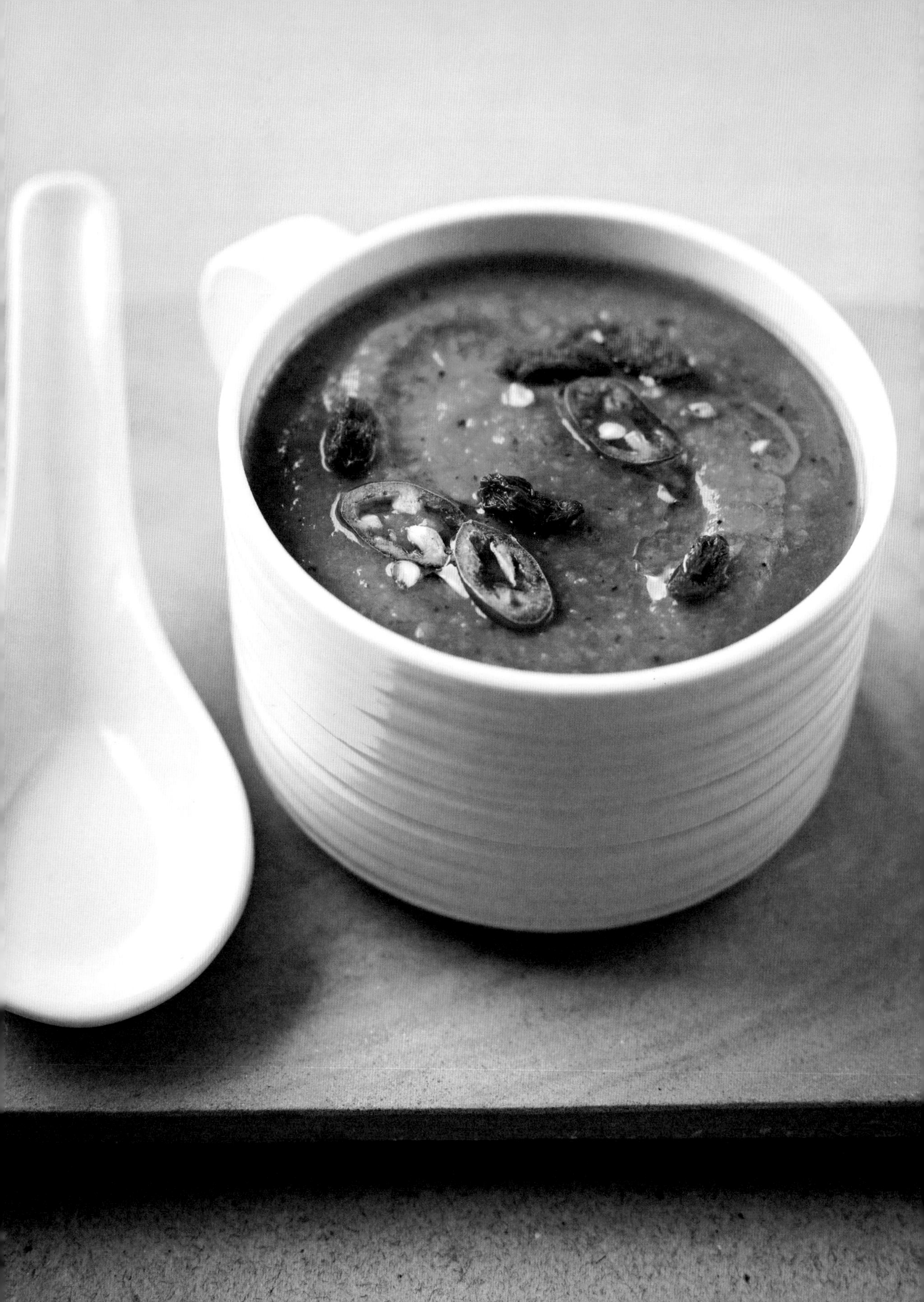

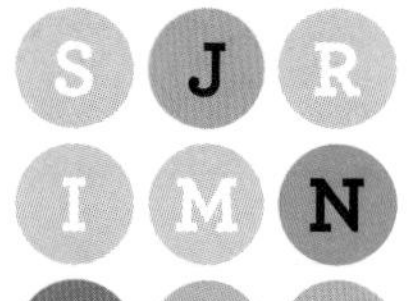

JOINTS & BONES *Arthritis*
MENTAL HEALTH & NERVOUS SYSTEM *Anxiety, Depression*
HEART & CIRCULATION *High cholesterol, High blood pressure*
DIGESTIVE SYSTEM *Bloating, Crohn's disease*
REPRODUCTIVE & URINARY SYSTEMS *Problematic periods*

Thai fish soup

This gorgeous dish has a lovely exotic vibe about it, is easy to make, plus it's light and bursting with nutrients. Does it get much better?

SERVES 3 TO 4

1 stalk fresh lemongrass
light olive oil, for cooking
½ red onion, finely minced
1 garlic clove, finely minced
½-inch piece fresh ginger, peeled and minced
2 kaffir lime leaves
1 14-ounce can coconut milk
2 salmon fillets (4 ounces each), skinned and cut into ½ inch cubes
6 ounces cooked shrimp
handful baby spinach leaves
3 ounces snow peas
juice of ½ lime
handful fresh cilantro leaves, torn
1 red chili pepper, thinly sliced (optional)

Bash the whole lemongrass stalk with something heavy, such as a rolling pin, to release the fragrant oils. Heat a little olive oil in a large pan, add the onion, garlic, ginger, kaffir lime leaves, and lemongrass and cook gently for 4 to 5 minutes, or until the onion has softened.

Add the coconut milk and ⅔ cup water, and cook at a slow simmer for 15 minutes. Add the salmon and continue to simmer until it is cooked—about 5 minutes.

Add the shrimp, spinach and snow peas and simmer for 2 more minutes. Squeeze in the lime juice, add the torn cilantro and chili pepper, remove the lemongrass stalk and lime leaves—and you're ready to serve. It's great with a side salad, or perhaps some noodles. You could add these to the soup along with the salmon (check the cooking time on the package).

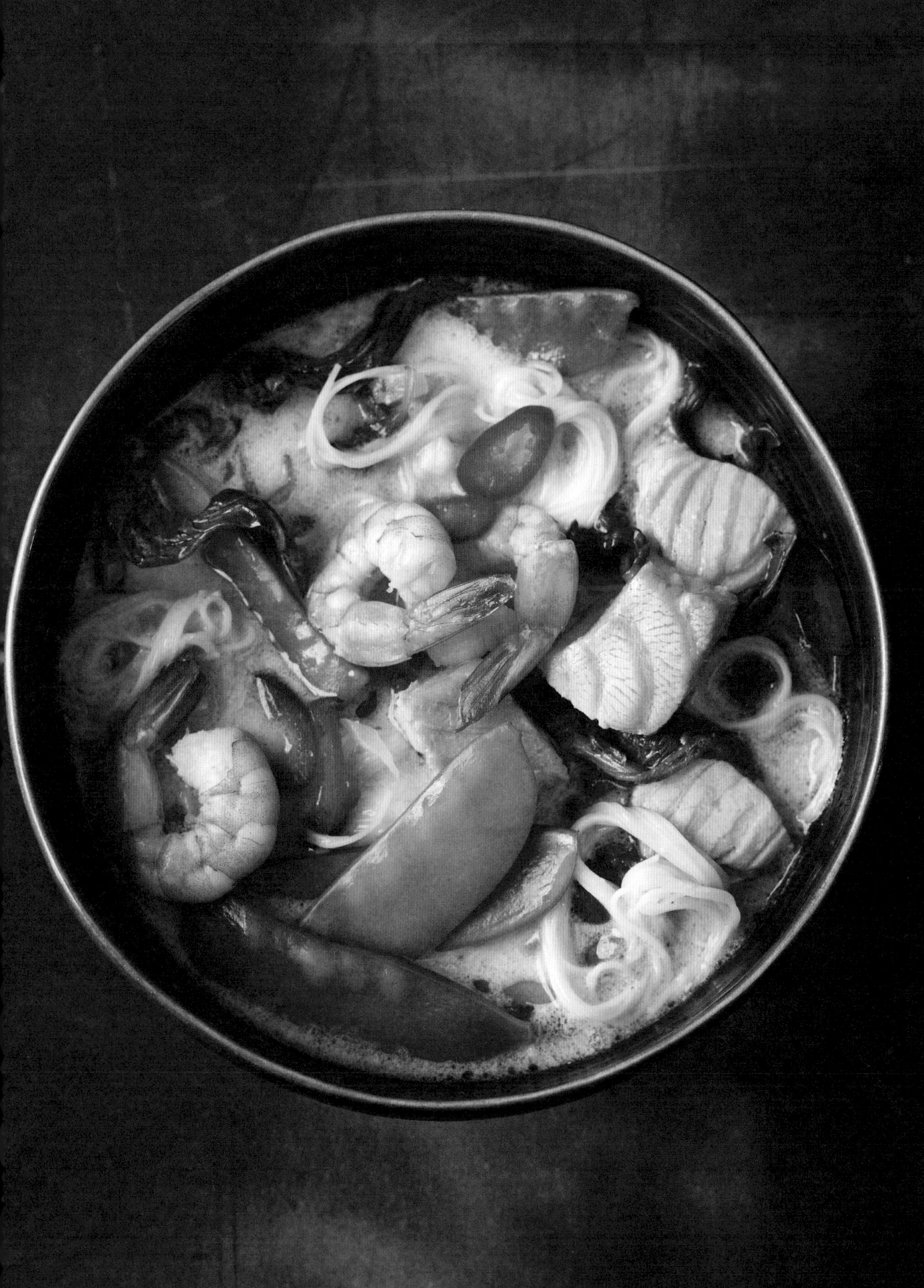

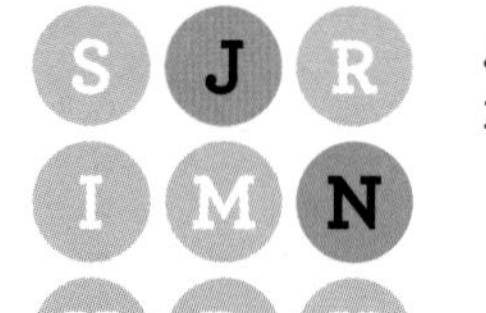

JOINTS & BONES *Osteoporosis, Rickets*
MENTAL HEALTH & NERVOUS SYSTEM *Anxiety*

Calming green soup

It's soup. It's green. That's for sure! This simple soup is not only an awesome color, but also has a naturally sweet flavor and a wonderfully smooth texture.

SERVES 3 TO 4

- olive oil, for cooking and drizzling
- 1 white onion, minced
- 1 garlic clove, minced
- 3 cups fresh or frozen peas
- 1 large zucchini, coarsely chopped
- 1 large potato, roughly diced, skin left on
- generous 2 cups vegetable stock (made from stock cubes or bouillon powder)
- 1 6-ounce bag baby spinach
- small bunch fresh mint leaves
- sea salt and black pepper

Heat a little olive oil in a large pan, add the onion and garlic, and cook for 4 to 5 minutes, or until softened.

Add the peas, zucchini, and potato, and enough vegetable stock to just cover all the ingredients. Simmer until the potato has softened, about 10 to 15 minutes.

Add the baby spinach a handful at a time, until it has all wilted into the hot soup. Add the mint leaves, setting aside a few small ones.

Season with salt and pepper. Transfer in batches to a blender and process to a smooth soup. Scatter with the reserved mint leaves and drizzle with a little olive oil to serve.

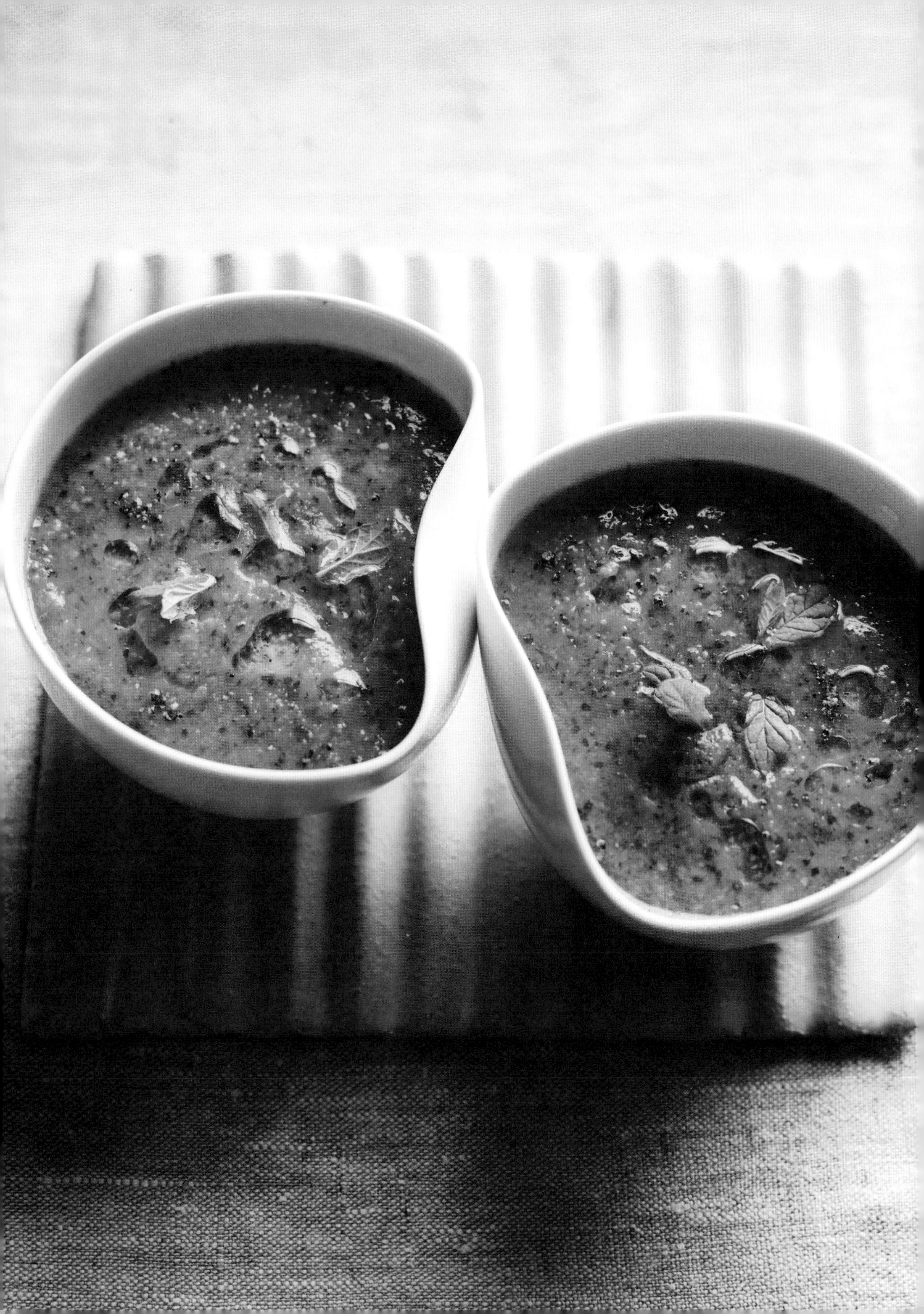

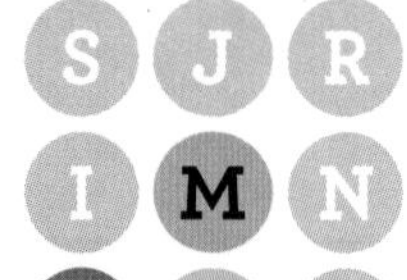

METABOLIC SYSTEM *Diabetes (Type 2)*
HEART & CIRCULATION *High cholesterol*
DIGESTIVE SYSTEM *Bloating*

Tomato and lentil soup

This is a wonderfully flavorful soup: ripe, fresh, and deep. You can even make a thicker version to use as a dip.

SERVES 3 TO 4

olive oil, for cooking
1 large red onion, minced
2 garlic cloves, minced
2 teaspoons ground cumin
1½ pounds cherry tomatoes
1 cup red lentils
4 cups vegetable stock (made with stock cubes or bouillon powder)
sea salt and black pepper
small bunch fresh parsley or cilantro, roughly chopped (optional)

Heat a little olive oil in a large pan, add the onion, garlic, and cumin, and cook over medium heat for 4 to 5 minutes, or until lightly golden.

Add the cherry tomatoes and cook over high heat, stirring frequently. Keep cooking until the tomatoes have started to turn into a bit of a mush, and the whole thing resembles a thick ratatouille.

Add the lentils and start adding the stock a little at a time, almost as though you're cooking a risotto. Each time the stock level goes down, add a little more. Keep doing this until the lentils are soft, about 15 to 20 minutes.

Once the lentils are soft, add enough stock to cover the whole mixture and season with salt and pepper. Transfer in batches to a blender and process to a smooth soup. Sprinkle with parsley or cilantro, if using, and serve immediately.

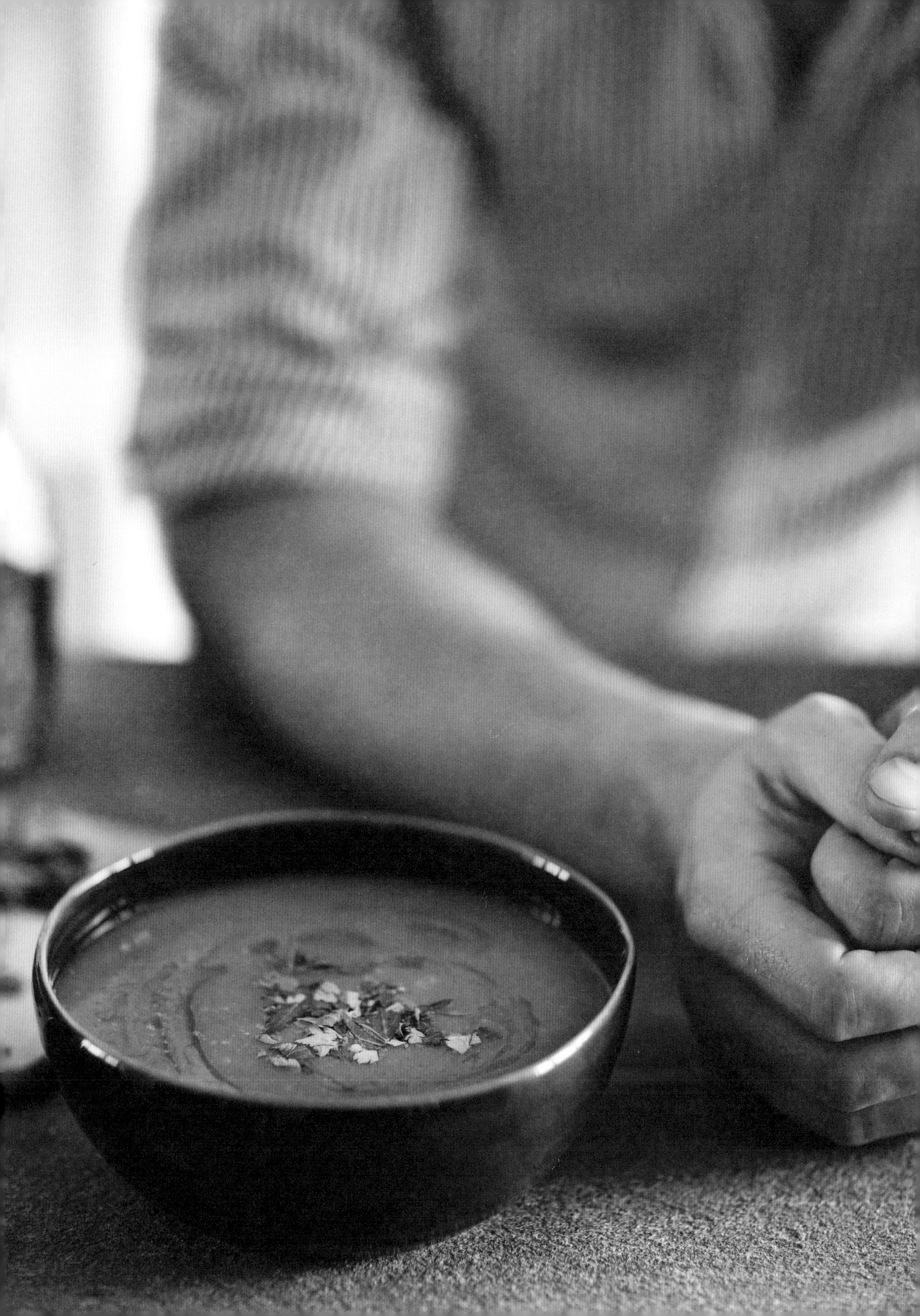

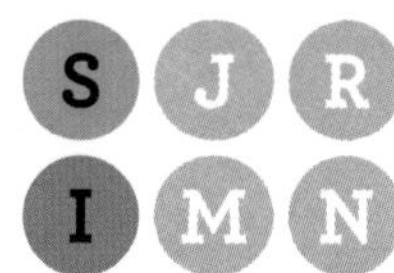
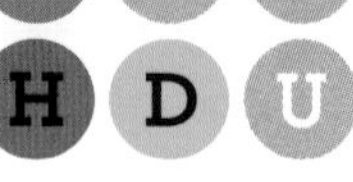

SKIN *Eczema*
IMMUNE SYSTEM
HEART & CIRCULATION *Heart disease, High blood pressure*
DIGESTIVE SYSTEM *Constipation*

Roasted butternut squash, garlic, and red lentil soup

This does take a bit of preparation, but it is totally worth it for the real depth of flavor. The roasting of the squash and the garlic brings out an intense, smoky sweetness that runs throughout the dish.

SERVES 4

- 1 large butternut squash, diced, seeded, skin left on
- 4 garlic cloves, left whole, with papery skin removed
- olive oil, for cooking
- sea salt and black pepper
- 1½ teaspoons dried mixed herbs
- ½ large red onion, minced
- 1¼ cups red lentils
- 3–4 cups vegetable stock (made with stock cubes or bouillon powder)
- 3–4 teaspoons green pesto (optional, Omega Pesto p 103)

Preheat the oven to 400°F. Place the diced butternut squash and garlic in a roasting pan, drizzle with olive oil, and sprinkle with salt and pepper and the dried herbs. Mix well and roast in the oven for 20 to 25 minutes, or until the squash is browning at the edges and the skin is crisp. The garlic will have turned a goldenish color, too.

Heat a little olive oil in a large pan, add the onion, and cook for 4 to 5 minutes, or until softened. Add the roasted squash, garlic, and lentils. Add enough vegetable stock to cover and simmer until the lentils are cooked.

Season with salt and pepper. Transfer in batches to a blender and process to a soup. Add a little more stock if the soup is too thick. Transfer to serving bowls and drizzle with a swirl of pesto in each bowl, if using. It's delicious served with toast topped with soft, fresh goat cheese.

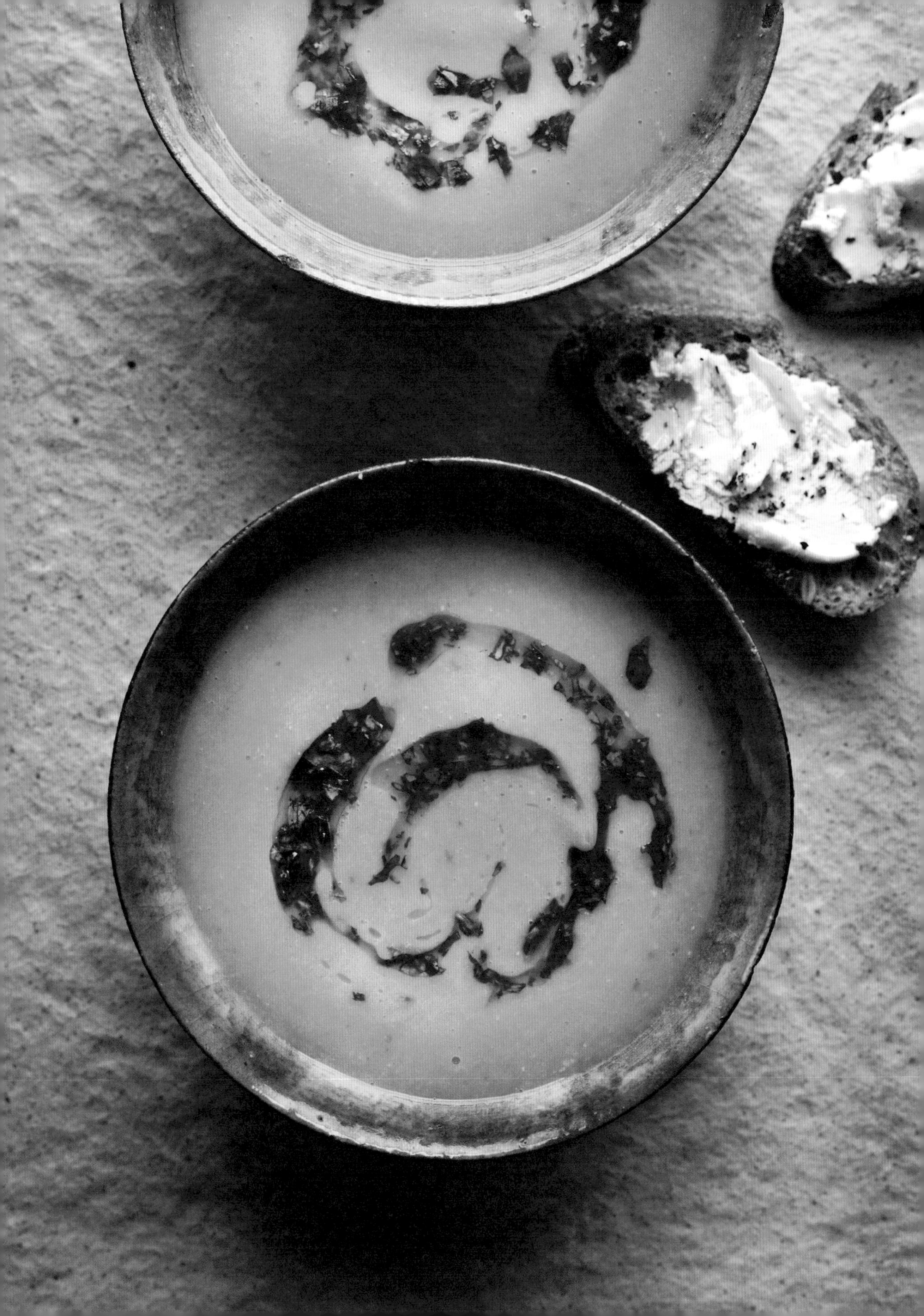

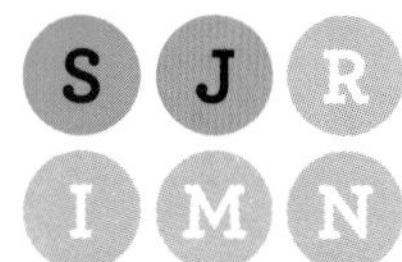
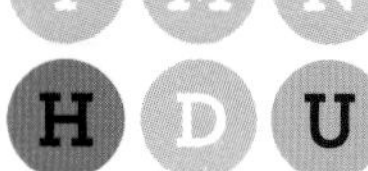

SKIN
JOINTS & BONES *Arthritis*
HEART & CIRCULATION *Heart disease*
REPRODUCTIVE & URINARY SYSTEMS *Prostate health*

Gazpacho

This beautiful cold soup is a real summer classic. It has a lovely Mediterranean vibe and bursts with flavor, and since it isn't cooked, it's incredibly rich in nutrients.

SERVES 2 TO 4

- 2¼ pounds very ripe tomatoes, coarsely chopped
- ½ small red onion, coarsely chopped
- 3 garlic cloves, coarsely chopped
- 1 cucumber, coarsely chopped
- 5 tablespoons olive oil, plus extra for drizzling
- 1 tablespoon red wine vinegar
- sea salt and black pepper

Put the tomatoes, onion, garlic, and cucumber in a blender, and blend at high speed for at least 1 minute, or until thoroughly puréed. If you like, you can set aside a little of the chopped red onion and cucumber to use as a garnish at the end.

Pass this mixture through a strainer, pushing it through the mesh with a wooden spoon. This will remove any coarse pulp and create a lovely, smooth mixture.

Put the strained mixture back into the blender and blend at the slowest speed. Add the olive oil and red wine vinegar slowly, to form a smooth, well-blended mixture. Season with salt and pepper.

Place in the refrigerator and chill well before serving. To serve, sprinkle with the reserved minced cucumber and onion, if using, and a drizzle of olive oil.

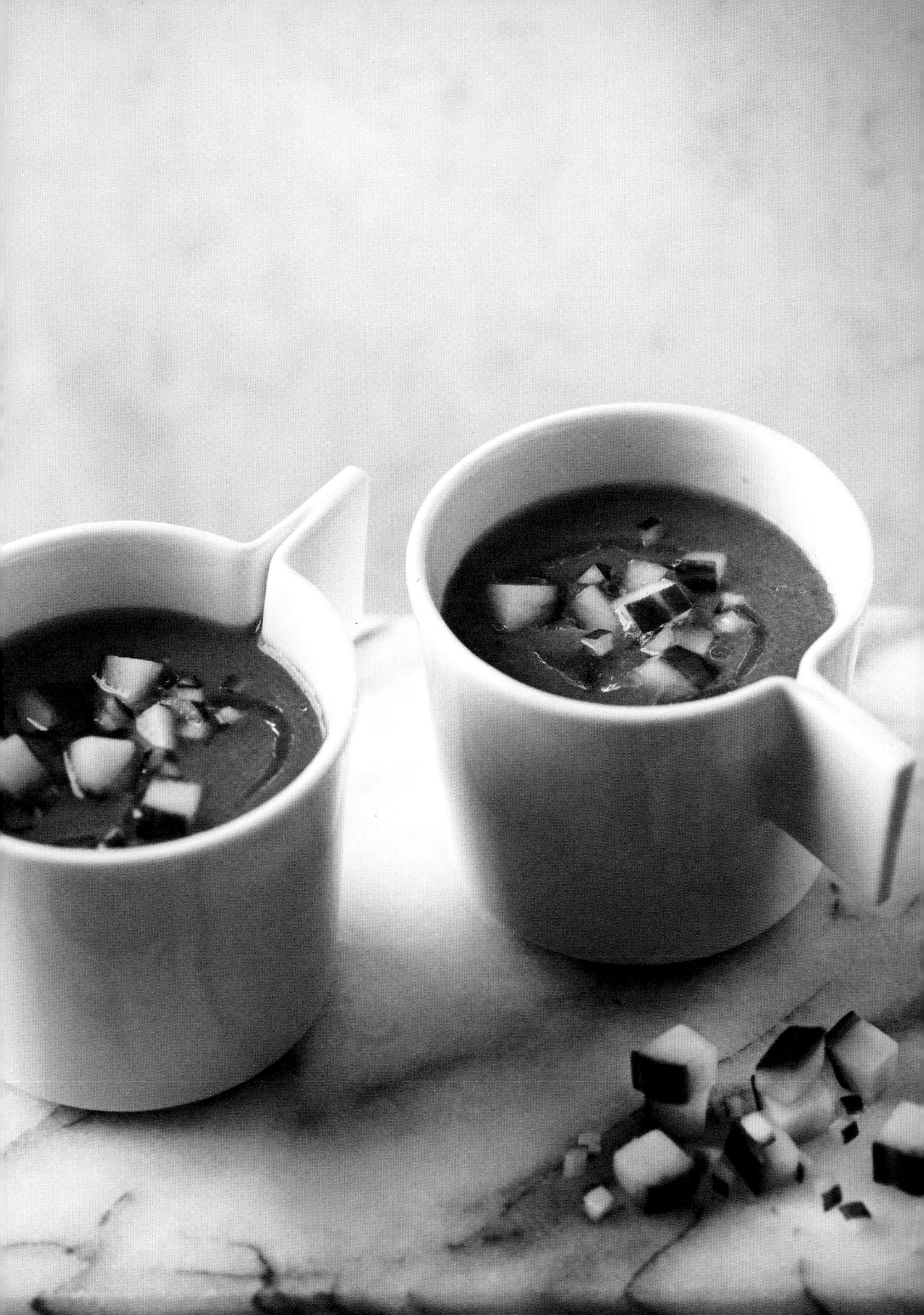

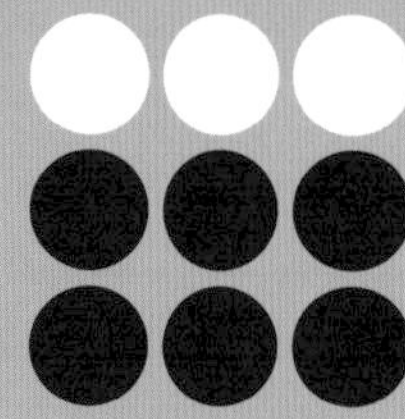

Light bites

There are often times when you want something light to nibble on—you might not feel like a full lunch or dinner, but you're peckish enough to need something. This is often when we reach for junk food, so I have devised some light bites that are perfect for moments like these.

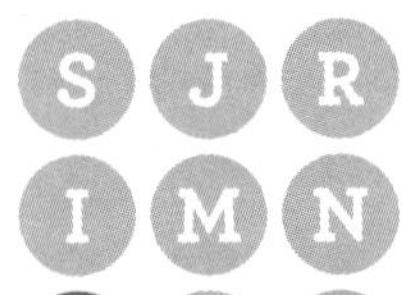

HEART & CIRCULATION *High cholesterol*
REPRODUCTIVE & URINARY SYSTEMS
Endometriosis, Menopause, Polycystic ovary syndrome, Problematic periods

Edamame and chickpea salad with lime, chili pepper, and cilantro

This is a wonderful salad that can make a really filling lunch, or a great side dish.

SERVES 2

1 14-ounce can chickpeas, drained
handful edamame beans, thawed if frozen
½ cucumber, diced
zest and juice of 1 lime
1 teaspoon honey
1 teaspoon light soy sauce
handful fresh cilantro leaves, finely chopped
1 large red chili pepper, sliced

Combine the drained chickpeas and edamame in a salad bowl, along with the diced cucumber.

Mix the lime zest and juice, honey, and soy sauce together to make a dressing.

Add the chopped cilantro and the dressing, and stir thoroughly. Top with the sliced red chili pepper and serve.

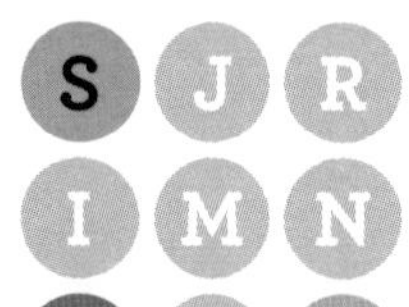

SKIN *Eczema, Psoriasis*
HEART & CIRCULATION *Heart disease, High blood pressure, High cholesterol*
REPRODUCTIVE & URINARY SYSTEMS *Prostate health*

Roasted vegetable and guacamole open sandwich This light little dish packs a mighty nutritional punch, and is very flavorful.

SERVES 1

½ red bell pepper, cut into ¾-inch chunks
½ red onion, thickly sliced
1 tablespoon extra-virgin olive oil, plus extra for drizzling
sea salt and black pepper
1 large, very ripe avocado
1 garlic clove, minced
1 small green chili pepper, minced
juice of ½ lime
2 slices whole grain bread, toasted

Preheat the oven to 400°F. Place the chopped bell peppers and onion in a small roasting pan. Drizzle with olive oil and season with salt and pepper. Roast in the oven for 15 to 20 minutes, or until the vegetables are soft and the onion is beginning to caramelize slightly at the edges.

Meanwhile, make the guacamole by scooping the flesh of the avocado into a food processor, along with the chopped garlic, chili pepper, 1 tablespoon olive oil and lime juice, and season with salt and pepper. Blend at full speed to create a smooth, creamy guacamole. If you prefer it chunky, mash the ingredients together in a bowl.

Place the slices of toast side by side on a plate, spread a generous helping of guacamole on each slice, and cover with the roasted vegetables. Serve immediately.

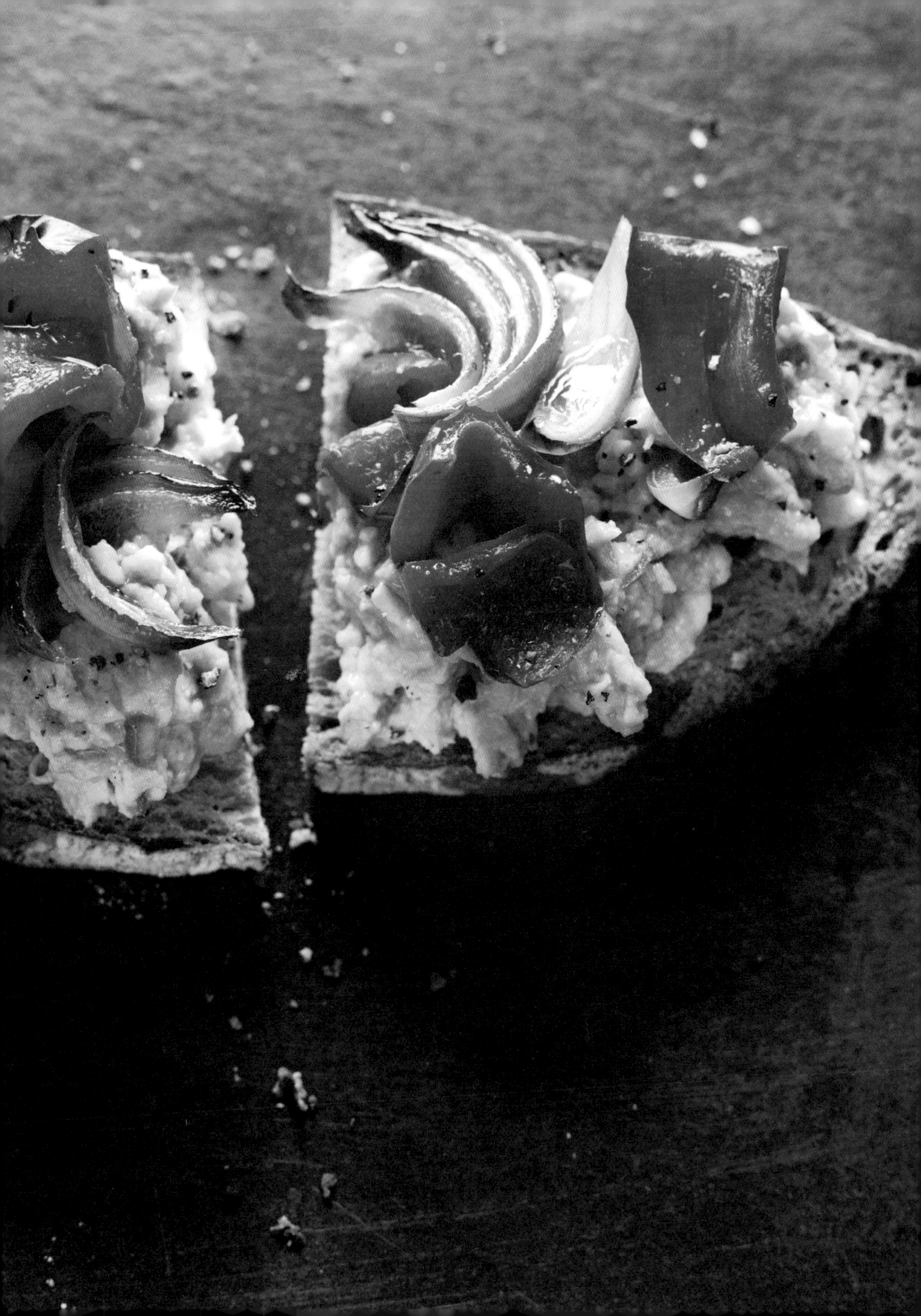

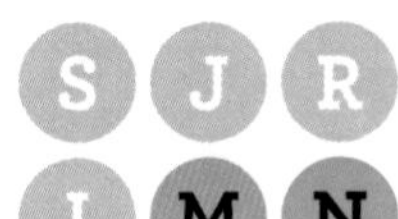
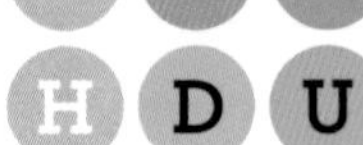

METABOLIC SYSTEM *Diabetes (Type 2)*
MENTAL HEALTH & NERVOUS SYSTEM *Stress*
DIGESTIVE SYSTEM
REPRODUCTIVE & URINARY SYSTEMS *Polycystic ovary syndrome*

Creamy egg on rye with wild arugula

This is so creamy and satisfying, and surprisingly filling for such a small dish.

SERVES 1

- 2 hard-boiled free-range eggs (see page 42), shelled
- 1 tablespoon live probiotic plain yogurt
- 1 small handful fresh chives, minced
- sea salt and black pepper
- 1 slice rye bread
- pinch of smoked paprika (optional)
- small handful wild arugula

Put the boiled eggs in a small bowl and mash them with the back of a fork to make a fine, crumbly mixture.

Add the yogurt and chives to the eggs, season with salt and pepper, and stir together to make a creamy egg spread.

Put a nice dollop of the egg spread on top of a slice of rye bread, and top with a little paprika and the wild arugula. Enjoy!

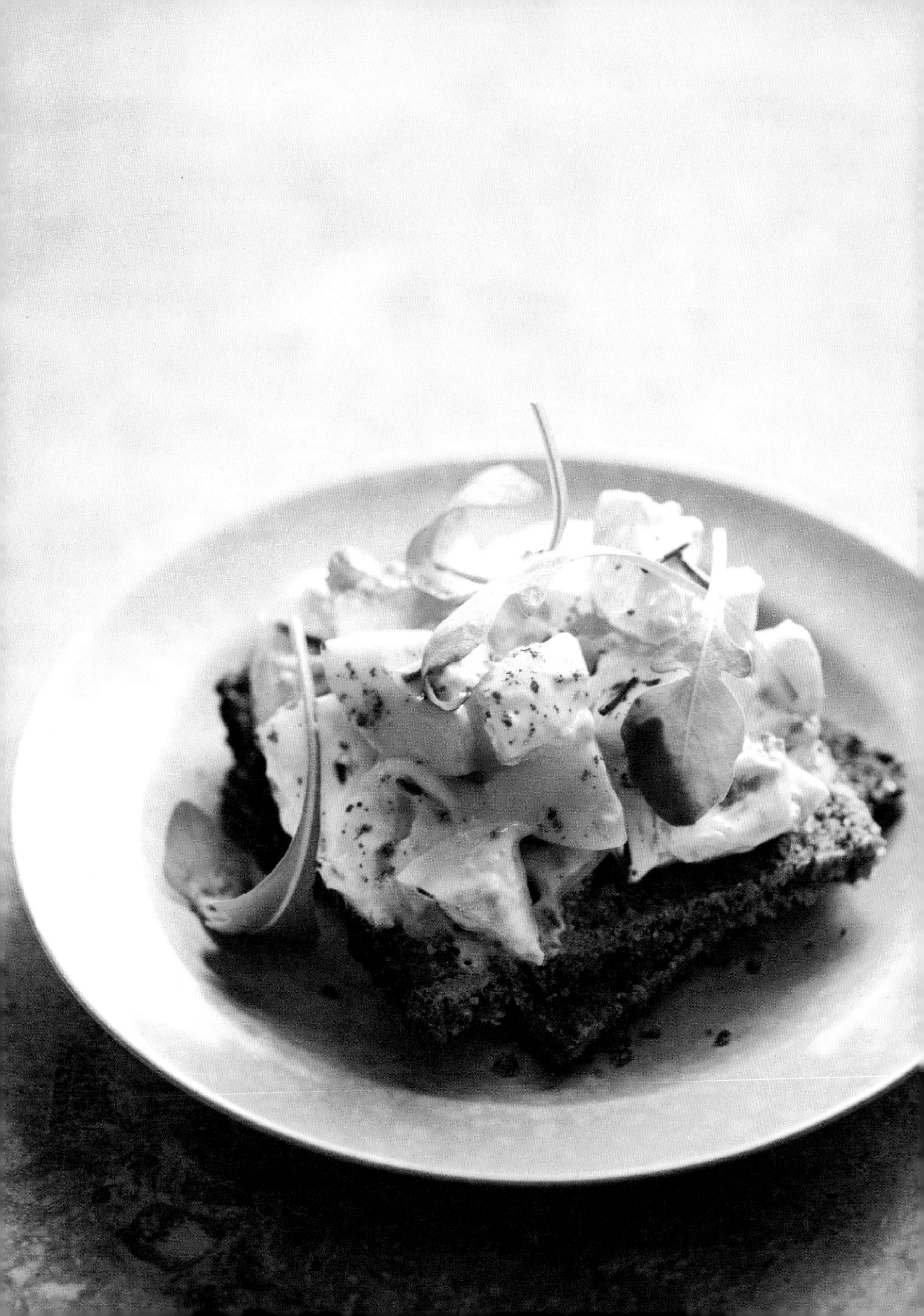

These recipes are major crowd-pleasers. The combination of olives and artichokes is bold, brassy, and will keep even the most hardened of healthy-food haters creeping back for more. Mint and feta is also a match made in heaven, and always conjures up images of the Mediterranean for me. I've used canned fava beans to save time, but by all means use fresh or frozen if you'd prefer.

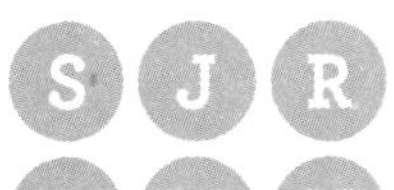
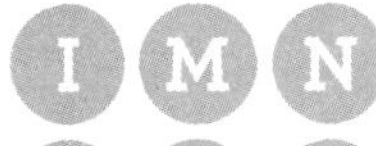

DIGESTIVE SYSTEM
Bloating

Fava bean, mint, and feta crostini

SERVES 2

1 11-ounce can fava beans, drained
small handful fresh mint leaves
3 tablespoons extra-virgin olive oil
¾ cup crumbled feta cheese
sea salt and black pepper

Place the beans, mint, and olive oil in a food processor and blend at low speed to create a coarse pâté. Transfer to a serving bowl.

Add the feta and stir gently to ensure there are small lumps of it throughout the pâté. Season with salt and pepper.

Serve the mixture on top of slices of toasted bread of your choice, such as a ciabatta, baguette, or sourdough.

SKIN
HEART & CIRCULATION
High cholesterol
DIGESTIVE SYSTEM
Constipation

Green olive and roasted artichoke crostini

SERVES 2 TO 3

1 12-ounce jar pitted green olives, drained, plus extra to garnish (optional)
1 12-ounce jar roasted artichoke hearts, drained
1 large garlic clove, coarsely chopped
3 canned anchovies, drained and roughly chopped (optional)
3 tablespoons olive oil
sea salt and black pepper

Put the ingredients in a food processor and process to a smooth paste. Season with salt and pepper.

Put a big dollop on a toasted slice of ciabatta, whole grain bread, a whole grain cracker, or anything else that floats your boat. Garnish with a few more olives, if desired.

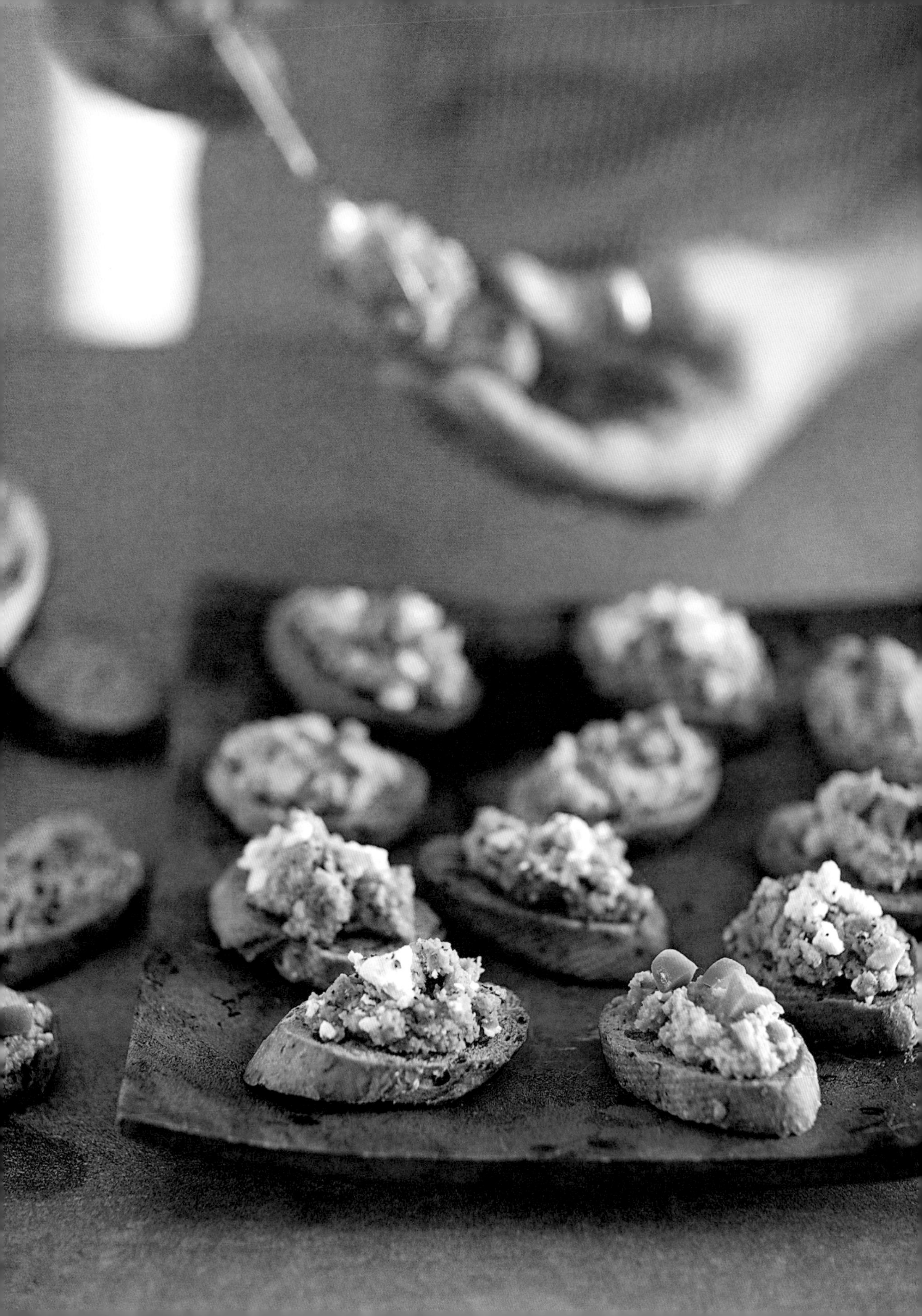

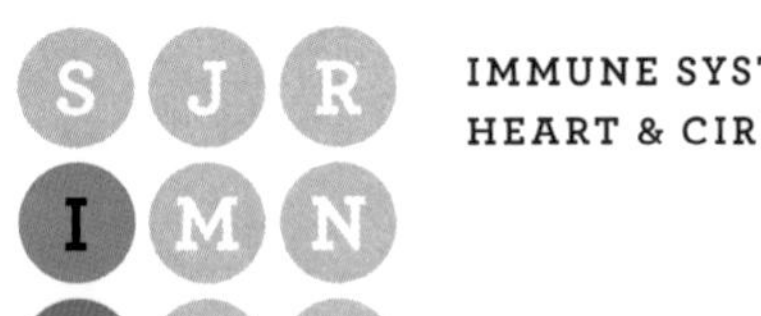

IMMUNE SYSTEM *Colds & flu*
HEART & CIRCULATION *High cholesterol*

Holy shiitake . . . pâté, that is! This is a lovely, earthy dish that's great on a whole grain cracker, used as a sandwich filler, or even as a dip for raw celery. It contains some seriously powerful active chemicals, too.

SERVES 3 TO 4

4 ounces raw shiitake mushrooms
scant ¾ cup sunflower seeds
1 garlic clove
2 teaspoons low-salt soy sauce

Put all the ingredients in a food processor and blend into a smooth pâté. Serve on crackers or whole wheat bread.

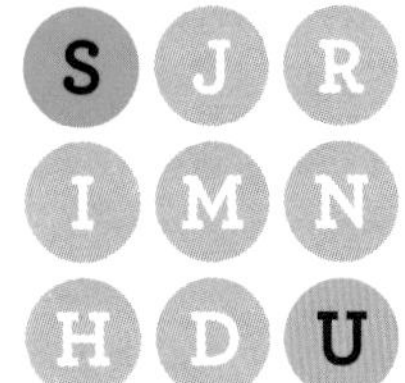

SKIN *Acne, Eczema*
REPRODUCTIVE & URINARY SYSTEMS
Polycystic ovary syndrome, Problematic periods

Walnut and watercress salad with blue cheese

I love this combo—the bold flavors and varied textures make it an interesting and pleasing dish. The creamy dressing with its slight peppery tones marries perfectly with the watercress and pungent blue cheese.

SERVES 2

scant 1½ cups bulgur wheat
½ cucumber, diced
1 cup cherry tomatoes, halved
1 cup walnuts
2 large handfuls fresh watercress
1 tablespoon mild horseradish sauce
3 tablespoons olive oil
sea salt and black pepper
½ cup crumbled blue cheese

Put the bulgur wheat in a pan and cover with freshly boiled water, then simmer over medium heat for 15 minutes, or until tender. Drain well.

Put the cooked bulgur wheat in a salad bowl. Add the cucumber, tomatoes, walnuts, and watercress, and stir well.

Mix together the horseradish and olive oil to make a creamy dressing, and season with salt and pepper.

Pour the dressing over the bulgur wheat and stir well. Scatter the blue cheese over the top and serve.

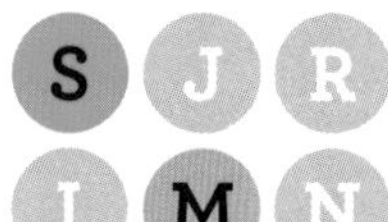
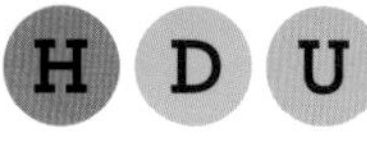

SKIN *Eczema*
METABOLIC SYSTEM *Diabetes (Type 2)*
HEART & CIRCULATION *Heart disease*
DIGESTIVE SYSTEM *Bloating, Constipation*
REPRODUCTIVE & URINARY SYSTEMS *Prostate health*

Greek pita pizza

This is my idea of a perfect feel-good snack. I am somewhat partial to proper pizza, and this treat makes the most of my favorite flavors.

SERVES 1

small handful baby spinach leaves
2–3 teaspoons tomato paste
1 large whole grain pita bread
½ garlic clove, minced
small sprig fresh mint leaves, coarsely torn
4–5 cherry tomatoes, halved if large
⅓ cup crumbled feta cheese
sea salt and black pepper
4 black olives, pitted

Begin by wilting the spinach. Place it in a pan with about 2 tablespoons freshly boiled water. Place over high heat so that the water simmers. Cover and cook for 3 to 4 minutes—the spinach will wilt very quickly. Remove from the heat, drain off any liquid, and let cool for a few moments. Once cool enough to handle, give it a squeeze to get rid of any excess water.

Preheat the broiler. Spread the tomato paste evenly over the pita bread. Add the minced garlic, wilted spinach, mint, cherry tomatoes, and feta. Season with salt and pepper and place the olives on top.

Place under the broiler for about 5 minutes, or until the cheese begins to get golden brown on the edges. Serve immediately.

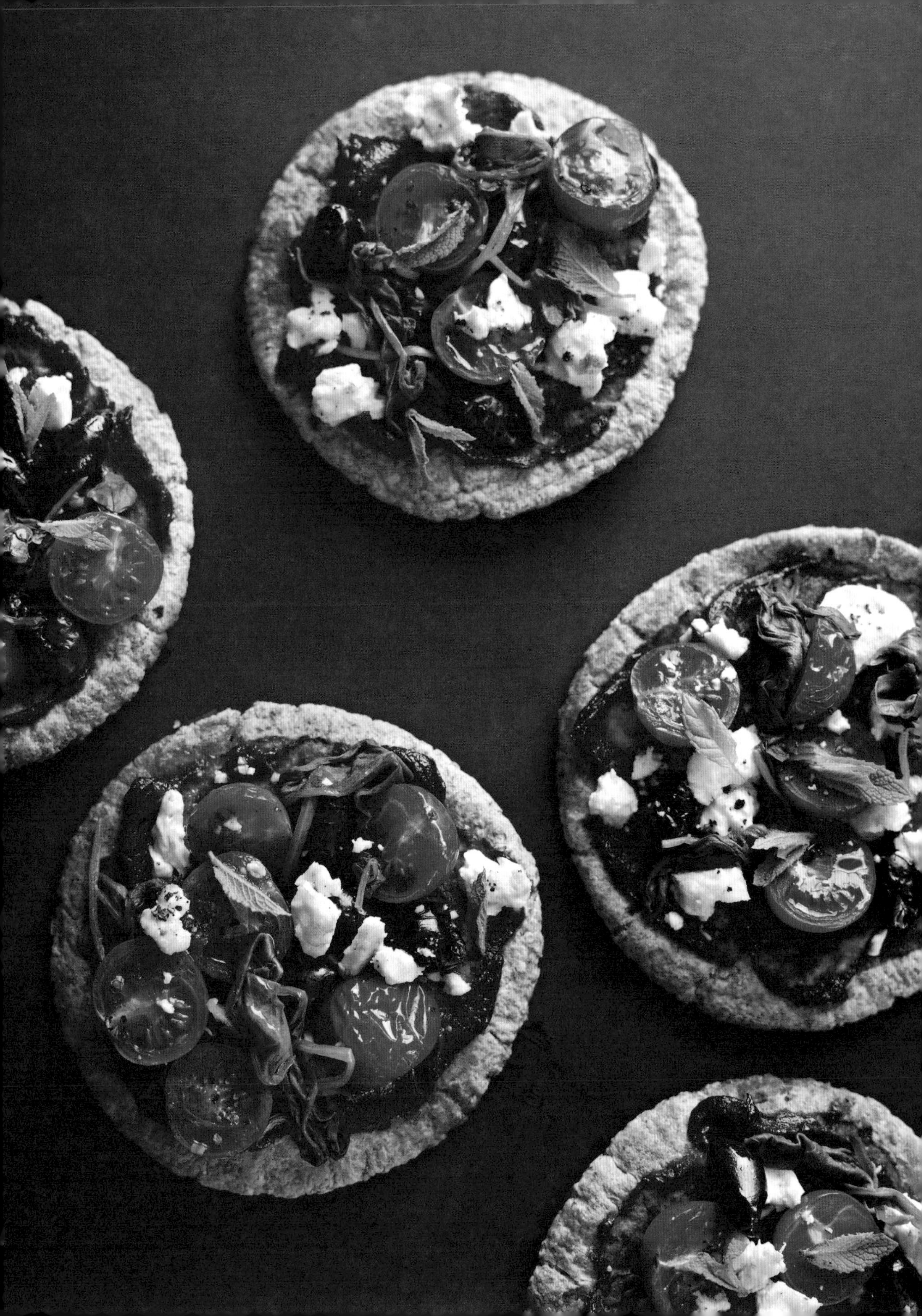

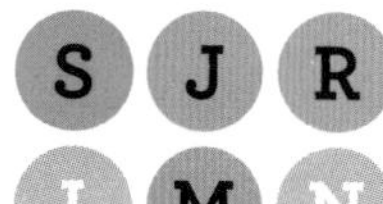
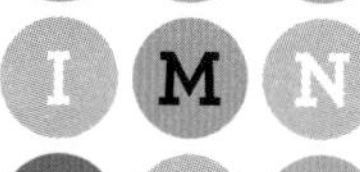
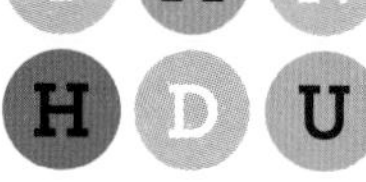

SKIN *Acne*
JOINTS & BONES *Osteoporosis*
RESPIRATORY SYSTEM *Asthma*
METABOLIC SYSTEM *Diabetes (Type 2)*
HEART & CIRCULATION *High blood pressure, High cholesterol*
REPRODUCTIVE & URINARY SYSTEMS *Problematic periods*

Heart-healthy tuna Niçoise salad

This is a wonderful, nutrient-dense salad, filled with flavor and very satisfying.

SERVES 1

handful baby spinach or mixed salad greens
5–6 raw green beans, thinly sliced lengthwise
2 large tomatoes, cut into wedges
1 hard-boiled free-range egg (see page 42), cut into quarters
6–7 black olives, pitted
5 canned anchovies, drained
olive oil, for cooking
1 fresh tuna steak, about 5 ounces

For the dressing:
2 tablespoons extra-virgin olive oil
1 teaspoon balsamic vinegar
sea salt and black pepper

Arrange the spinach, beans, tomato wedges, boiled egg wedges, and olives on a plate. Place the anchovies over the top in a circular pattern.

Heat a grill pan or skillet with a little olive oil over medium-high heat. Add the tuna steak and cook for about 3 minutes on each side, so that it's still slightly pink in the middle. Don't move it around while cooking, apart from turning it over once. Remove from the heat.

Combine the dressing ingredients and season with salt and pepper. Slice the tuna into ¼-inch thick slices, and arrange the slices on top of the salad. Drizzle the dressing over the salad and serve.

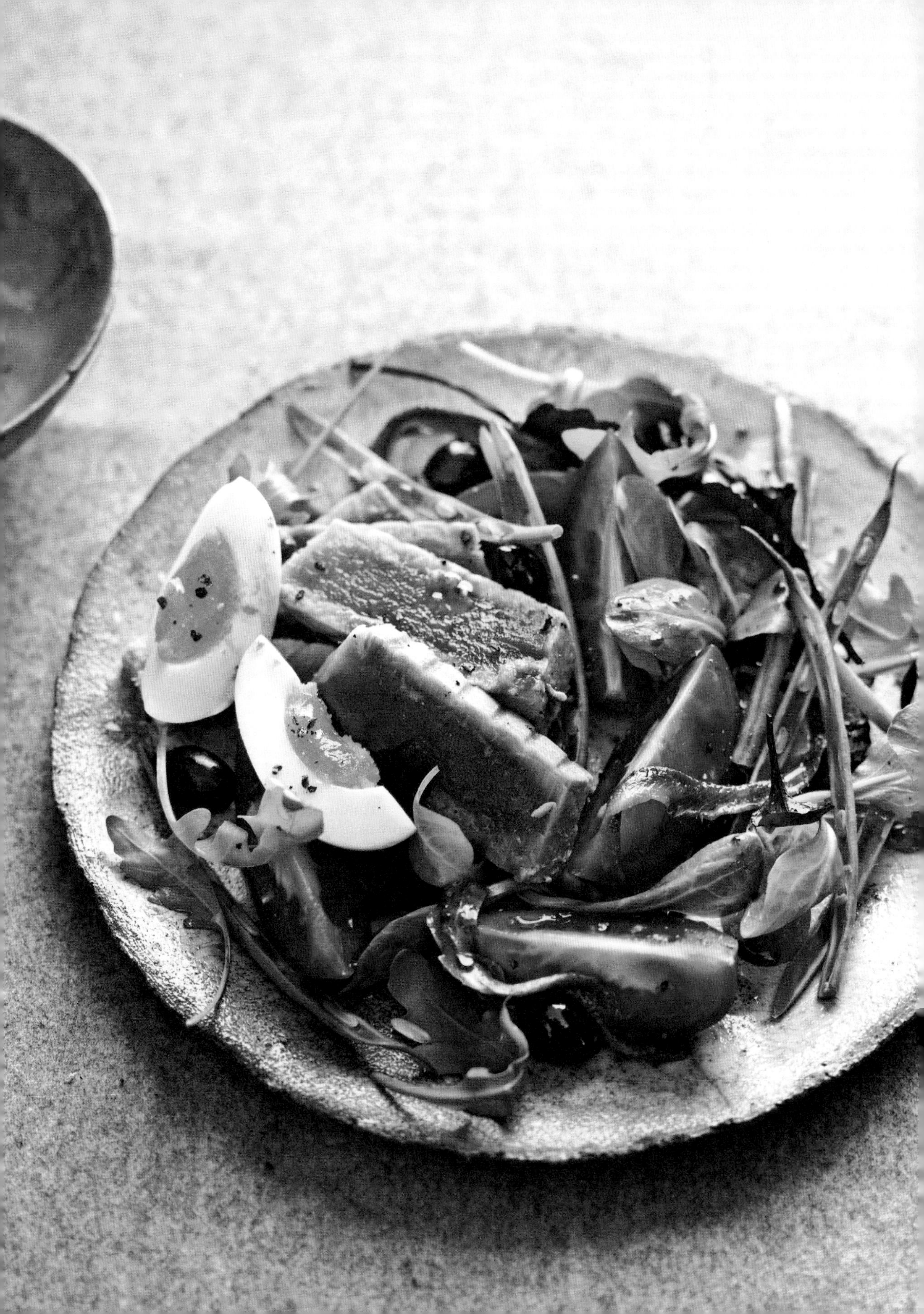

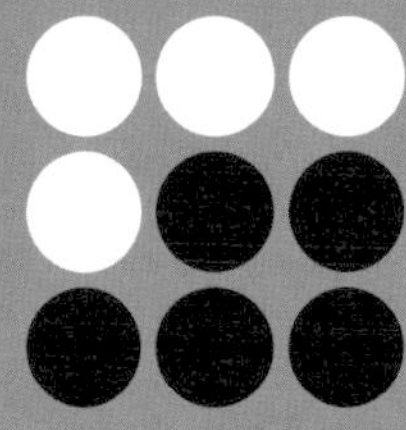

Small plates, sides & sharing

When we get together and want some food for sharing, we so often reach for junk. But you can still stick to your good eating habits and make an impressive platter to enjoy with your friends. These recipes have been designed to be suitable as appetizers or side dishes, or dishes that can be shared, tapas or mezze-style

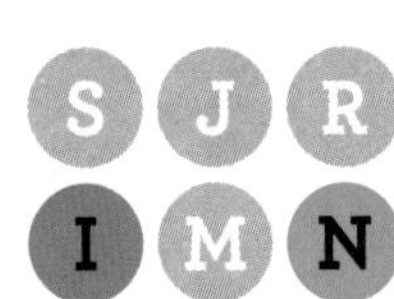

IMMUNE SYSTEM *Colds & flu*
MENTAL HEALTH & NERVOUS SYSTEM *Anxiety, Stress*
HEART & CIRCULATION *Heart disease, High blood pressure, High cholesterol*
DIGESTIVE SYSTEM

Stir-fried satay greens

This dish is a total dynamo. I got a well-known radio host addicted to it and she now eats it several times a week! When you taste it, I think you'll know why.

SERVES 1 TO 2

- olive oil, for cooking
- 1 large leek, sliced into thin rings
- 2 garlic cloves, finely sliced
- 1 small green or red chili pepper, minced (if you don't like it too spicy, you can discard the seeds)
- 2 handfuls shredded greens, such as napa cabbage, bok choy, and tatsoi
- about 1 tablespoon dark soy sauce
- 2 teaspoons honey
- 2 tablespoons good-quality crunchy peanut butter (no added salt or sugar)
- ½ teaspoon Chinese five-spice powder
- sea salt

Heat a little olive oil in a wide, shallow pan or wok and add the leek, garlic, and chili pepper. Cook for 5 to 8 minutes over medium heat, or until the leek is soft.

Add the shredded spring greens and continue to cook until they have softened slightly and turned a brighter green.

Add 2 dashes of soy sauce (about 1 tablespoon), the honey and the peanut butter, and stir well. Sprinkle the Chinese five spice over and stir again. Season with salt, if needed, and serve immediately. It's great with brown rice or a fillet of white fish.

Edamame beans make a wonderfully zingy dip that's great as an accompaniment to almost anything, such as vegetable crudités, pita bread, or corn chips—the works! My variation on red pepper hummus also goes with everything, but skips roasting the bell peppers, thereby keeping the nutrients intact.

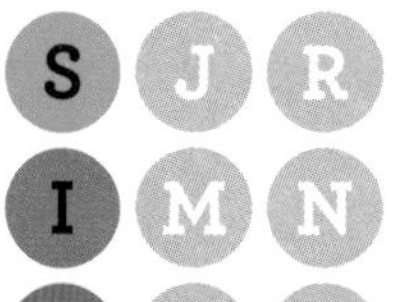

SKIN *Acne, Eczema*
IMMUNE SYSTEM *Colds & flu*
HEART & CIRCULATION *High cholesterol*

Red bell pepper and white bean dip

SERVES 2 TO 4

2 red bell peppers, diced
1 14-ounce can cannellini beans, drained
1 garlic clove, minced
2 tablespoons extra-virgin olive oil
sea salt and black pepper

Put the bell peppers, garlic, olive oil, and cannellini beans (except for 1 tablespoon of the beans) into a food processor. Season with salt and pepper and process to make a thick, luscious dip. Stir the reserved beans through the dip and serve with sliced toasted pita bread, celery sticks, or any other suitably "dippy" ingredient.

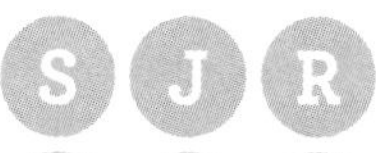

I M N
H D U

HEART & CIRCULATION *High cholesterol*
REPRODUCTIVE & URINARY SYSTEMS *Endometriosis, Menopause, Problematic periods*

Edamame dip with green chili pepper and garlic

SERVES 2–4

1½ cups fresh or frozen shelled edamame, thawed if frozen
1 garlic clove, minced
1 green chili pepper, minced
1–2 tablespoons extra-virgin olive oil
sea salt and black pepper

Put all the ingredients into a food processor, season with salt and pepper, and process to make a smooth dip. Serve with your choice of things to dip.

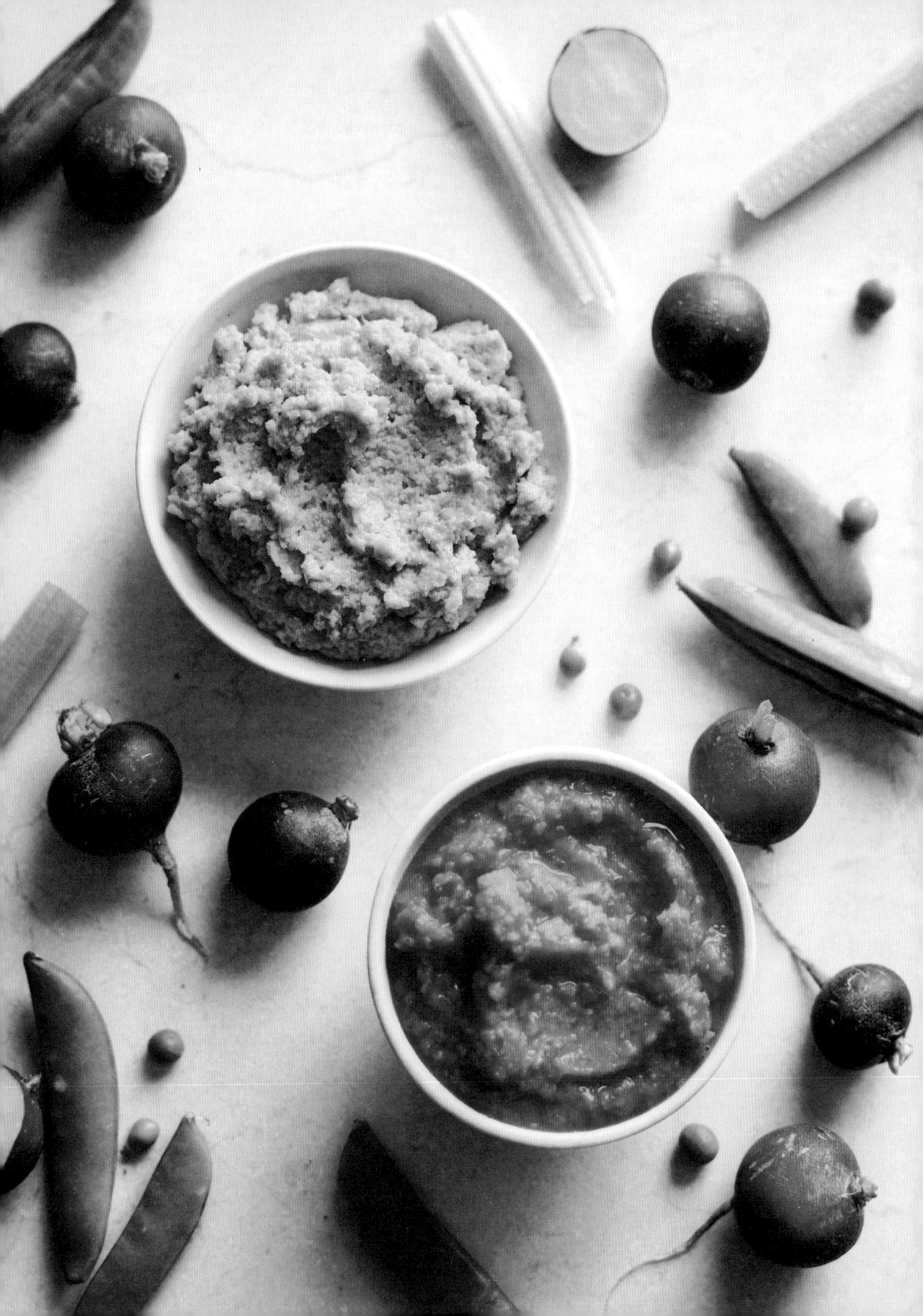

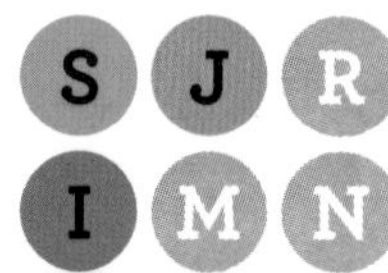

SKIN *Eczema*
JOINTS & BONES *Bursitis*
IMMUNE SYSTEM *Colds & flu*
HEART & CIRCULATION *Heart disease, High cholesterol*
DIGESTIVE SYSTEM *Hemorrhoids*

Purple power salad

This does exactly what it says on the can: it's purple and powerful! The compounds that make plants purple have many effective properties. I use flaxseed oil for its high omega 3 content. It's easy to find in your local health food store, and you could swap it for olive oil if you prefer.

SERVES 2

¼ red cabbage, finely grated
½ red onion, finely grated
1 large or 2 small raw red beets, finely grated
2 tablespoons flaxseed oil
1 teaspoon honey
1 teaspoon balsamic vinegar
½ garlic clove, minced
1 teaspoon toasted sesame seeds
sea salt and black pepper

Mix the red cabbage, red onion, and red beets together in a large serving bowl. Combine the flax seed oil, honey, and balsamic vinegar in a small bowl. Add the garlic. Stir well and drizzle over the grated vegetables.

Sprinkle with toasted sesame seeds and season with salt and pepper. Mix together thoroughly and serve. If you like, you can prepare the dressing in advance and mix it with the vegetables just before serving.

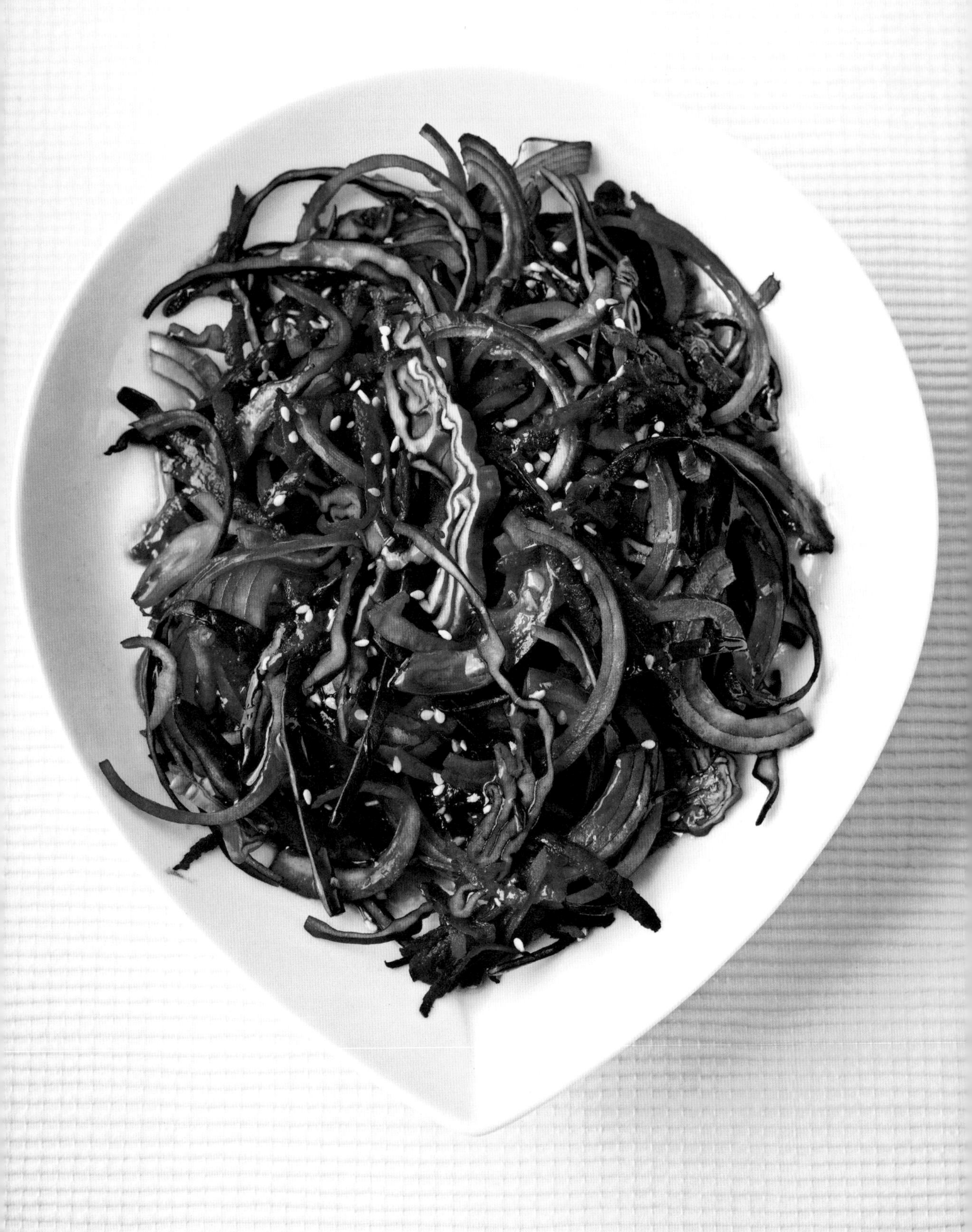

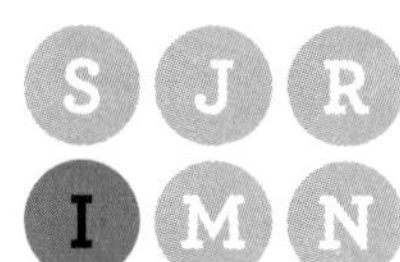

IMMUNE SYSTEM *Colds & flu*
HEART & CIRCULATION
DIGESTIVE SYSTEM

Dynamite dip

This dip has a wonderful, punchy, peppery flavor. It creates a powerful kick for the taste buds and ramps up digestion too!

SERVES 2 TO 4

- 1 14-ounce can lima beans, drained
- large handful watercress
- 1 garlic clove, minced
- 1 tablespoon extra-virgin olive oil
- sea salt and black pepper
- 2 large pita breads, cut into fingers

Preheat the broiler. Put the lima beans, watercress, garlic, and olive oil into a food processor and process to make a smooth purée. Season with salt and pepper.

Put the pita fingers on a baking sheet and toast under the broiler for a couple minutes, turning once, until crisp and toasted. Serve with the dip.

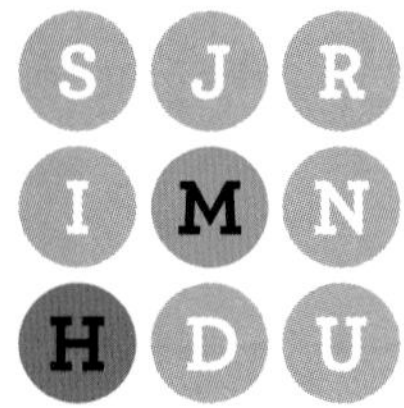

METABOLIC SYSTEM *Diabetes (Type 2)*
HEART & CIRCULATION *Heart disease*

Soft goat cheese, red onion, and chili spread

Goat cheese is lighter and much better tolerated by most people than cow's milk cheese. Its lovely, tangy flavor gets my mouth watering every time. The added bonus is that the fats in the cheese help with absorption of some of the beneficial compounds in the onions.

SERVES 2 TO 4

½ cup soft goat cheese
1 tablespoon olive oil
1 teaspoon red wine vinegar
¼ red onion, minced
½ green chili pepper, minced
small bunch fresh parsley leaves, minced
sea salt and black pepper

Put the goat cheese in a bowl, add the rest of the ingredients, and season with salt and pepper. Stir until all the ingredients are well combined. Serve with whole grain crackers or crudités.

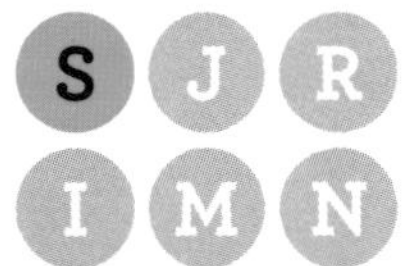

SKIN *Eczema, Psoriasis*
HEART & CIRCULATION *Heart disease, High blood pressure*
DIGESTIVE SYSTEM *Constipation*

Roasted red beet wedges with avocado and horseradish

This is the most amazing combination of flavors, and is sure to become a dinner-party favorite. It really is a match made in heaven.

SERVES 2 TO 4

- 4 large red beets, trimmed but unpeeled, and cut into wedges
- 2 tablespoons olive oil, plus extra for drizzling
- 2 large, ripe avocados
- juice of ½ lemon
- 3–4 teaspoons prepared horseradish
- sea salt

Preheat the oven to 400°F. Place the red beet wedges on a baking sheet, drizzle with olive oil, and season with salt. Roast in the oven for 20 to 25 minutes, or until soft. Let cool.

Peel the avocados. Make the sauce by putting the avocado flesh, lemon juice, horseradish, and olive oil into a food processor. Season with salt and blend into a smooth sauce to serve with the beets. This dish is great with a substantial side salad or some cooked couscous.

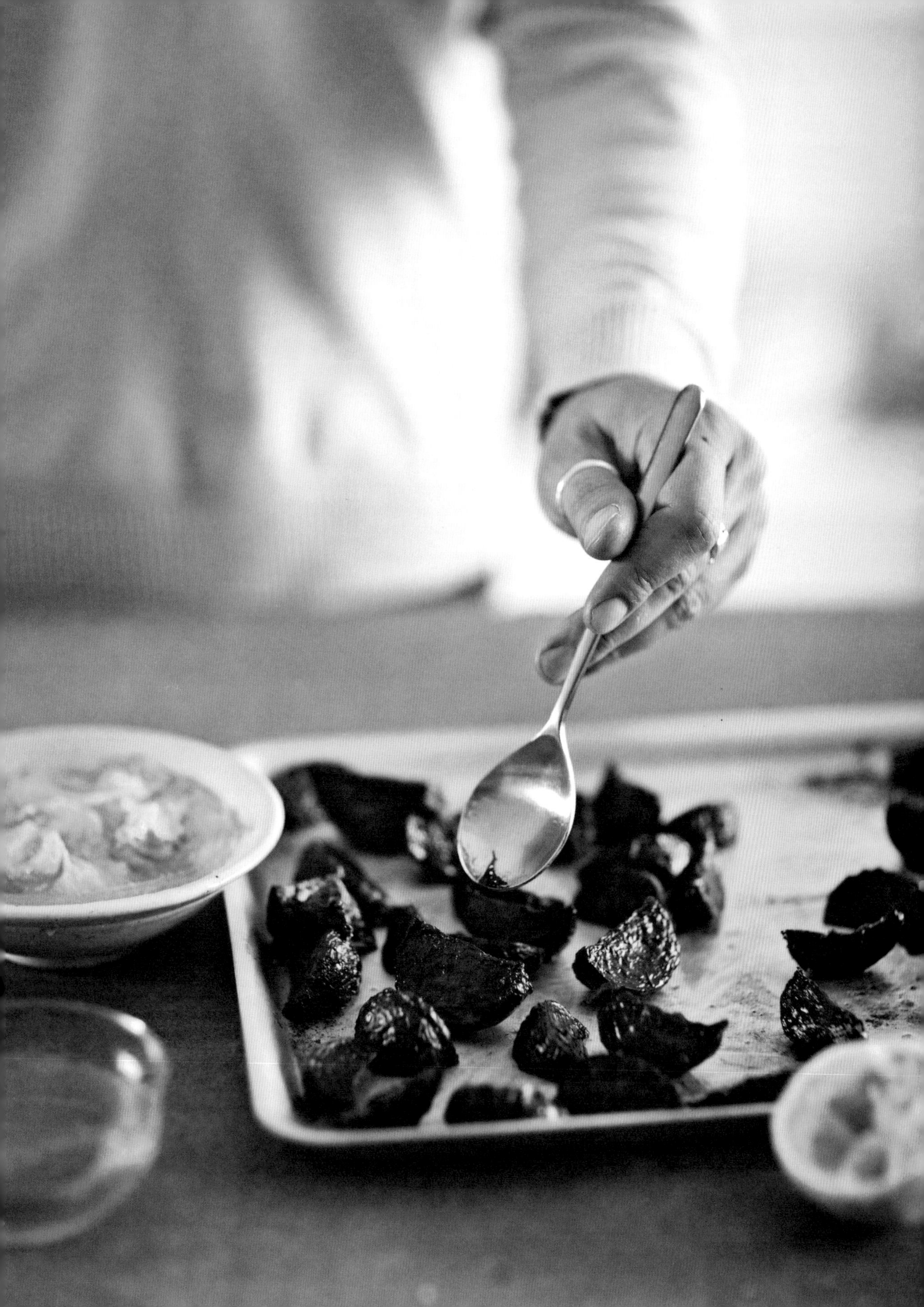

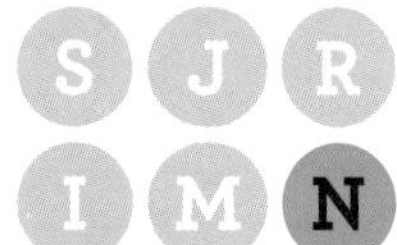

MENTAL HEALTH & NERVOUS SYSTEM *Anxiety*
HEART & CIRCULATION *High cholesterol*
DIGESTIVE SYSTEM *Constipation*
REPRODUCTIVE & URINARY SYSTEMS
Endometriosis, Polycystic ovary syndrome, Problematic periods

Garlicky white beans with kale and Parmesan

This is the ultimate comfort food for me. It's incredibly flavorful, creamy, and just really bakes my cookie! It's easy to make and is very potent. It works as a simple meal or a side dish.

SERVES 4 TO 6

- olive oil, for cooking
- 2 garlic cloves, thinly sliced
- 1 14-ounce can cannellini beans, drained
- 1 14-ounce can lima beans, drained
- large handful curly kale
- sea salt and black pepper
- 2 tablespoons grated Parmesan cheese
- ¼ teaspoon red pepper flakes (optional)

Heat a pan with a little olive oil and add the garlic. Cook over medium-high heat—this is one of those rare occasions that I encourage you to let the garlic go brown. This gives the dish a unique, smoky flavor.

At this point, add the beans and tear in the curly kale (tear it into small pieces straight into the pan). Season with salt and pepper. Continue to cook for 7 to 8 minutes, or until kale is just tender but still crisp.

At this stage, add 1 tablespoon of the Parmesan and stir well. Transfer to a serving dish and sprinkle the remaining Parmesan on top, along with some red pepper flakes, if using. Serve immediately.

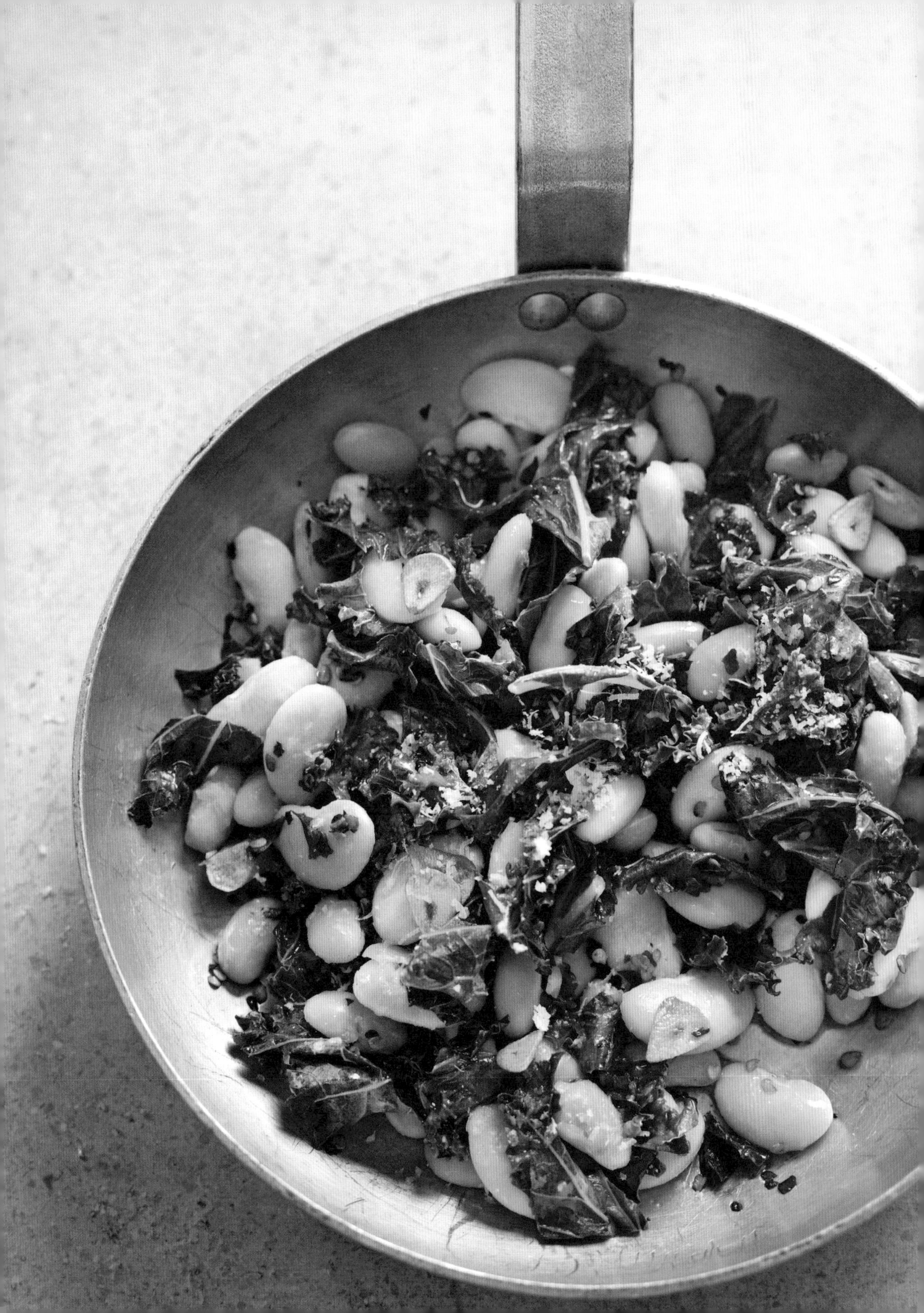

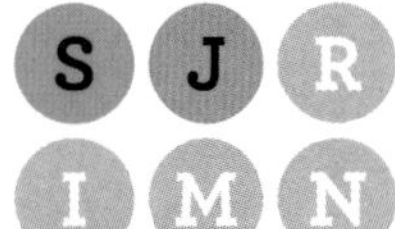

SKIN *Acne, Eczema, Psoriasis*
JOINTS & BONES *Arthritis*
HEART & CIRCULATION *Heart disease*
DIGESTIVE SYSTEM *Crohn's disease*

The beta booster

I love the intense, earthy, and aromatic flavors in this dish. The squash is ultrarich in the antioxidant beta-carotene, and the fats in the feta cheese actually drastically increase the body's absorption of the beta-carotene.

SERVES 4

- 1 medium butternut squash
- 3 garlic cloves
- 1 teaspoon cumin seeds
- ¼ teaspoon red pepper flakes
- olive oil, for roasting
- small bunch fresh sage, finely minced, or 1 teaspoon dried sage
- sea salt
- 1½ cups crumbled feta cheese
- black pepper

Preheat the oven to 400°F. Halve the butternut squash, scoop out the seeds, and discard them. Dice the squash (keeping the skin on) into ½-inch cubes. Place these in a roasting pan.

Keep the garlic cloves whole and unpeeled. Bash them with the palm of your hand or the back of a wooden spoon—anything that will partially crush them. Add them to the roasting pan with the squash, and sprinkle over the cumin seeds and red pepper flakes. Drizzle over some olive oil, season with salt, and if you are using dried sage, add it at this point.

Roast in the oven for around 20 minutes, or until the squash is soft, starting to brown, and the edges are starting to caramelize. If using fresh sage, sprinkle it over now.

Place the squash in a large bowl and spinkle the feta over it, then season with a little black pepper. Serve immediately.

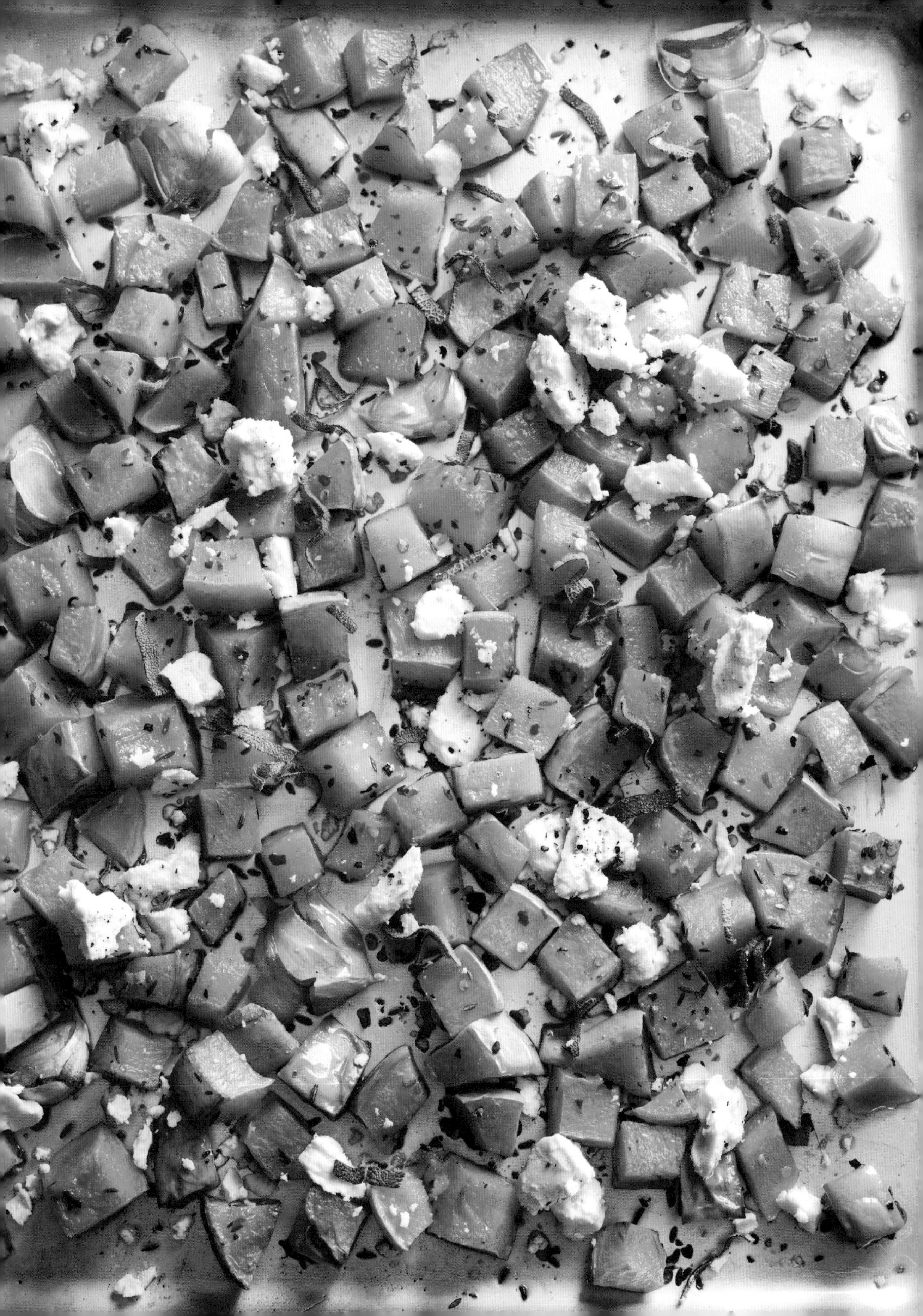

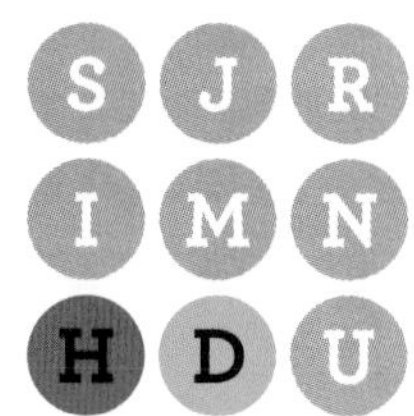

HEART & CIRCULATION *High blood pressure, High cholesterol*
DIGESTIVE SYSTEM *Constipation*

Spicy coconut dal

This is a fantastic fusion dish. It has the texture and appearance of a traditional Indian dal, but the inclusion of lemongrass gives it a Thai-Malay twist, and the end result is a true Asian fusion. Warning—this dish is addictive!

SERVES 3 TO 4

2 fresh lemongrass stalks
olive oil, for cooking
1 large red onion, minced
2 garlic cloves, minced
1 green chili pepper, minced
½ cup red lentils
¾ cup coconut milk
1¾ cups hot vegetable stock (made with a stock cube or bouillon powder)
sea salt and black pepper
small bunch fresh cilantro leaves, roughly chopped
1 red chili pepper, thinly sliced (optional)
1 lime, cut into wedges

Start by bashing the lemongrass. Use a rolling pin or something with plenty of weight behind it—this will split and bruise the stalk and allow the wonderful fresh oils to seep out of the lemongrass and into the dish.

Heat a little olive oil in a large pan, add the onion, garlic, chili pepper, and lemongrass and cook for 4 to 5 minutes, or until the onion has softened. Add the lentils and coconut milk and simmer for 3 to 4 minutes.

Start adding the vegetable stock, little by little. Keep adding the stock until the lentils have softened and partially broken down, which usually takes about 20 to 25 minutes.

Season with salt and pepper, sprinkle over the cilantro and red chili pepper, and serve immediately with the lime wedges on the side. It's great with quinoa with some goji berries, fresh cilantro, and lime juice stirred through it.

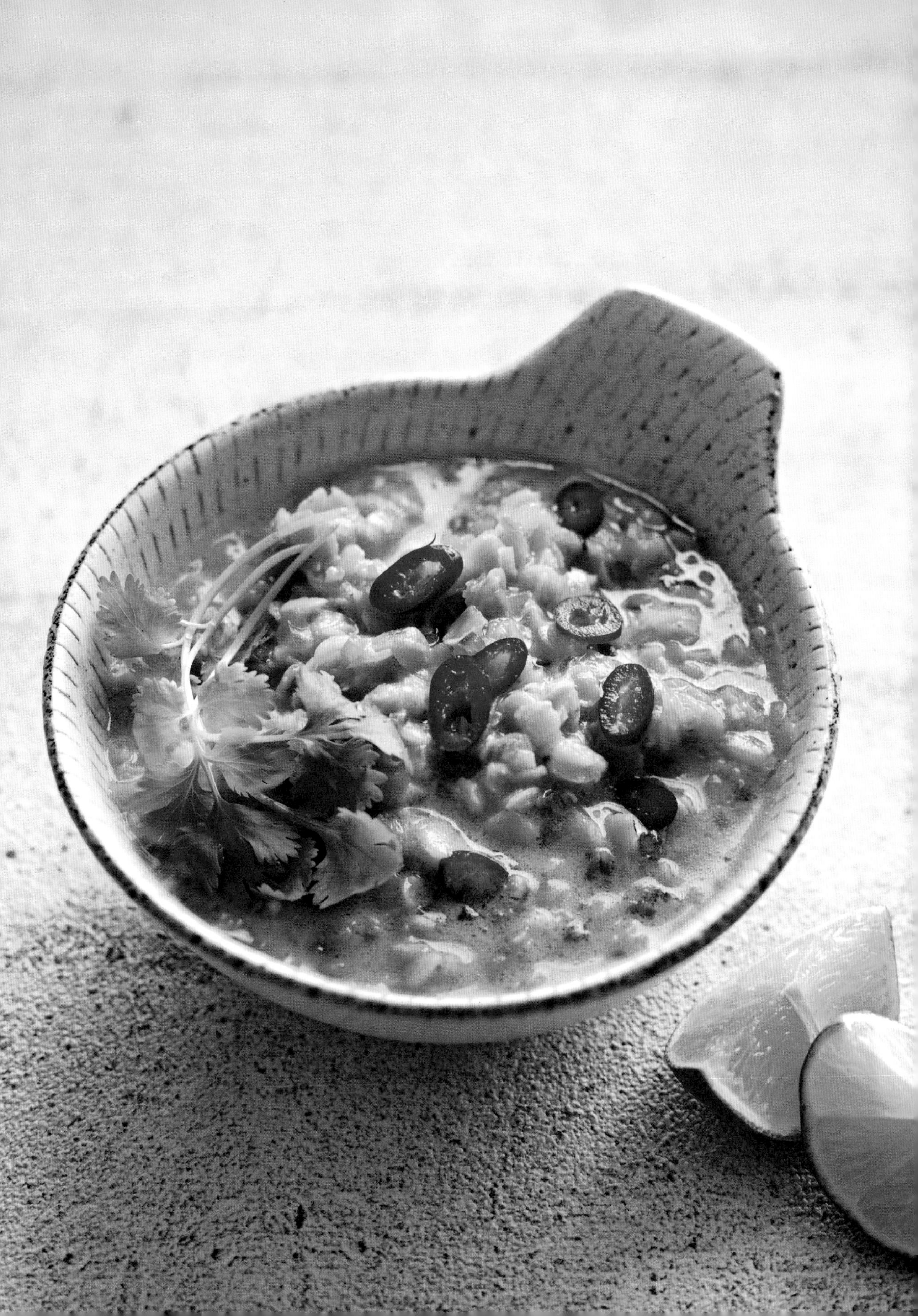

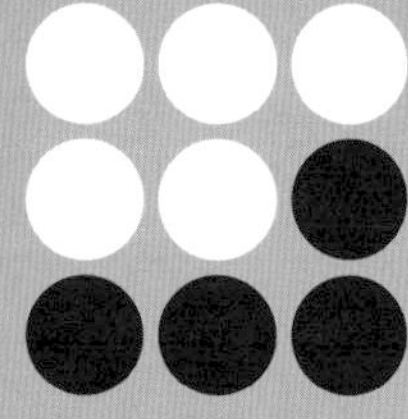

Handy, healthy snacks

Snacking is often a problem when we're trying to eat well. Temptation is everywhere and convenience is paramount, so it's all too easy to reach for a chocolate bar, a bag of potato chips, or other such undesirable items. However, with a bit of planning and organization, you can make some simple, handy snacks that will both scratch that itch for something to nibble on, and be nutritionally sound too. These are some of my favorites.

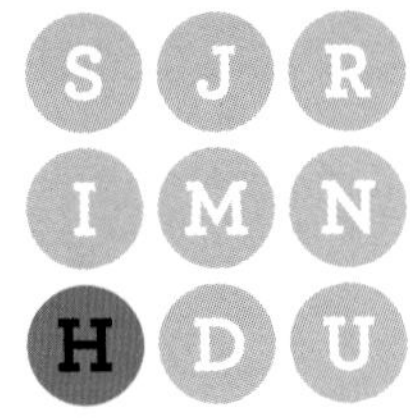

Delectable date slices

Date slices are sweet, gooey, incredibly addictive, and made my way are actually pretty good for you, providing a great general energy boost.

SERVES 6 TO 8

2/3 cup pitted dates, choppd
5 ounces coconut oil, plus extra for greasing
3 tablespoons honey
Scant 1 cup rolled oats
Scant 1¼ cups whole wheat flour
3 tablespoons mixed seeds

Preheat the oven to 300°F and grease an 8-inch square baking pan with coconut oil. Place the dates in a pan with 4 tablespoons water. Place the pan over low heat, cover, and cook the dates for a minute or two, until they form a gooey paste.

In another pan, melt the honey and coconut oil.

In a bowl, mix together the oats, flour, and mixed seeds. Pour in the melted honey and coconut mixture and stir well to form a dough.

Spoon half the dough into a greased baking pan, pushing down firmly. Top with the date mixture, and then spread the remaining dough over the date mixture.

Bake in the oven for about 30 minutes, or until golden brown. Let cool completely before cutting into squares.

These are great little dishes to have on hand in the refrigerator for those times when you want to dip into something tasty. They are rich in flavor, feel luxurious, and do you good at the same time. Guacamole is a fantastic comfort food that's full of the good fats that are vital for virtually every system in your body.

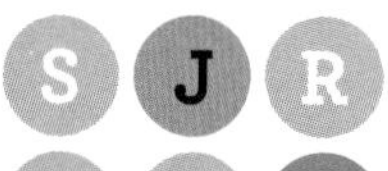

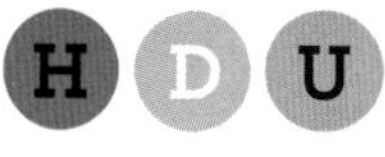

JOINTS & BONES
Osteoporosis
MENTAL HEALTH & NERVOUS SYSTEM
Anxiety, Stress
HEART & CIRCULATION
High blood pressure, High cholesterol
REPRODUCTIVE & URINARY SYSTEMS
Problematic periods

Stress-free smoked mackerel pâté

SERVES 2 TO 3

3 smoked mackerel fillets
3 tablespoons live probiotic plain yogurt
sea salt and black pepper
juice of ½ lemon
1 tablespoon capers, drained and roughly chopped

Flake the mackerel fillets into a food processor, discarding the skin. Add the yogurt and lemon juice, and season with salt and a generous helping of black pepper.

Process at slow speed, then stir in the capers, setting aside a few to sprinkle over the top. If you prefer a coarser texture, you can mash it with a fork instead. Serve it with vegetable crudités.

SKIN *Psoriasis*
HEART & CIRCULATION
Heart disease

Skin-boosting guacamole

SERVES 1 TO 2

2 large, very ripe avocados
2 tablespoons extra-virgin olive oil
juice of ½ lime
1 garlic clove, minced
1 fresh green chili pepper, minced
sea salt
¼ large red onion, minced
5–6 cherry tomatoes, quartered
black pepper

Halve the avocados and scoop out the flesh into a food processor. Add the oil, lime juice, garlic, and chili pepper, along with a good pinch of salt, and process on full power to make a smooth purée. If you don't have a food processor or prefer a coarser texture, you can mash the ingredients together with a fork.

Transfer the guacamole to a bowl. Add the chopped onion and tomatoes, and stir well. Season with salt and black pepper, and it is ready to serve.

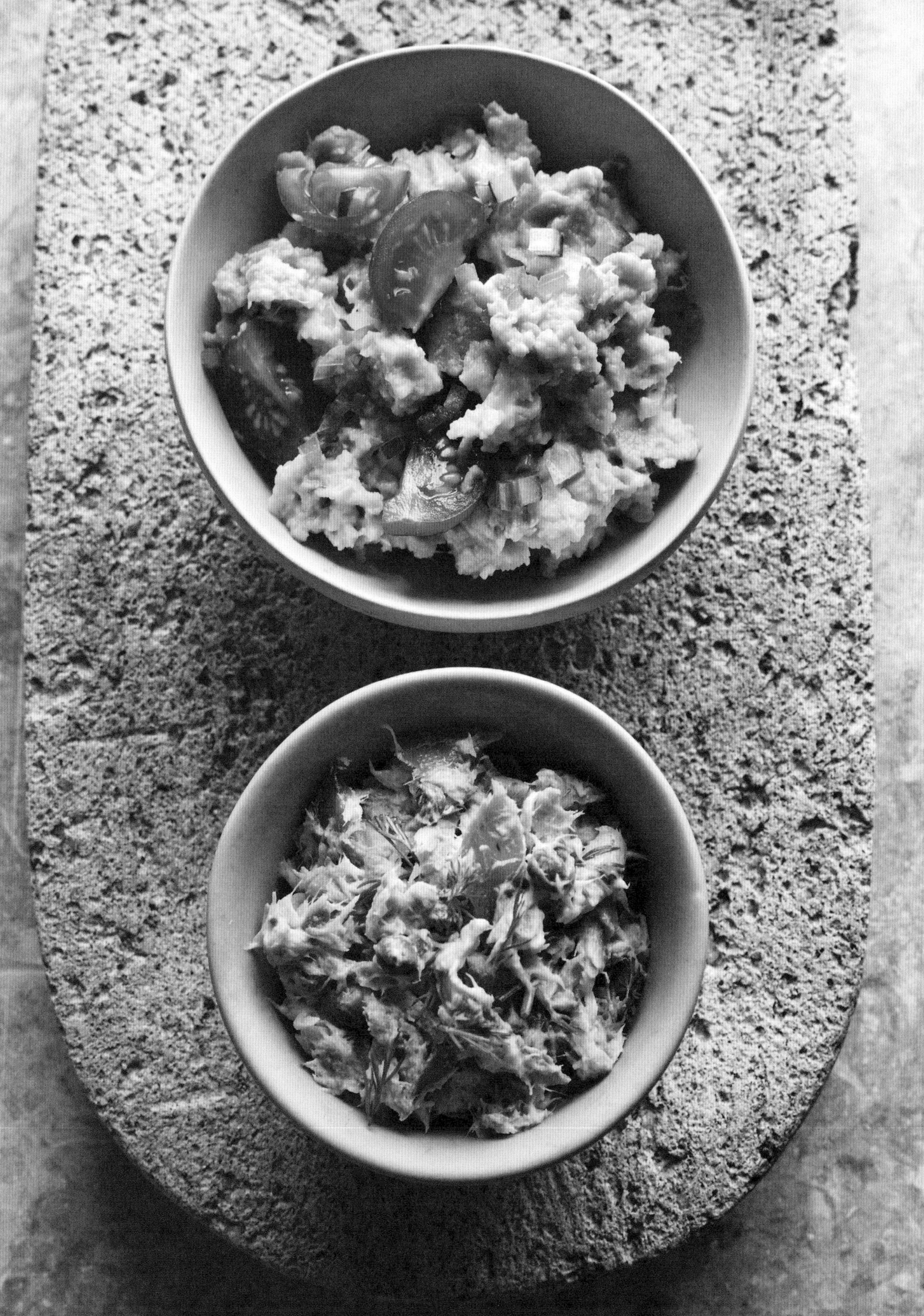

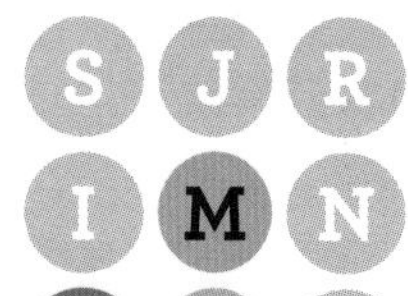

METABOLIC SYSTEM *Diabetes (Type 2)*
HEART & CIRCULATION *High cholesterol*
DIGESTIVE SYSTEM *Constipation, Hemorrhoids, IBS*

Apple and cinnamon oat squares These have the most fantastic, moist texture. The combination of cinnamon with oats is always a winner with me.

MAKES 6 TO 10 SQUARES

- 2 tablespoons coconut oil, plus extra for greasing
- 2 apples
- 2 tablespoons honey
- generous 2 cups rolled oats
- 2 teaspoons cinnamon
- 1 tablespoon dried cranberries (optional)
- 1 tablespoon pumpkin seeds (optional)

Preheat the oven to 350°F and grease an 8-inch square baking pan with coconut oil. Cut the apples into quarters, remove the seeds, then place them, unpeeled, in a food processor. Process to a coarse purée, adding a splash of water if necessary.

Melt the coconut oil and honey together in a pan over medium-high heat. Once the oil and honey have combined, add the apple purée and stir well.

Add the oats, cinnamon, cranberries, and pumpkin seeds and stir thoroughly to form a sticky mixture.

Transfer the mixture to the prepared pan, pressing down well, and bake for about 20 minutes, or until the top is golden brown. Let cool completely before cutting into squares.

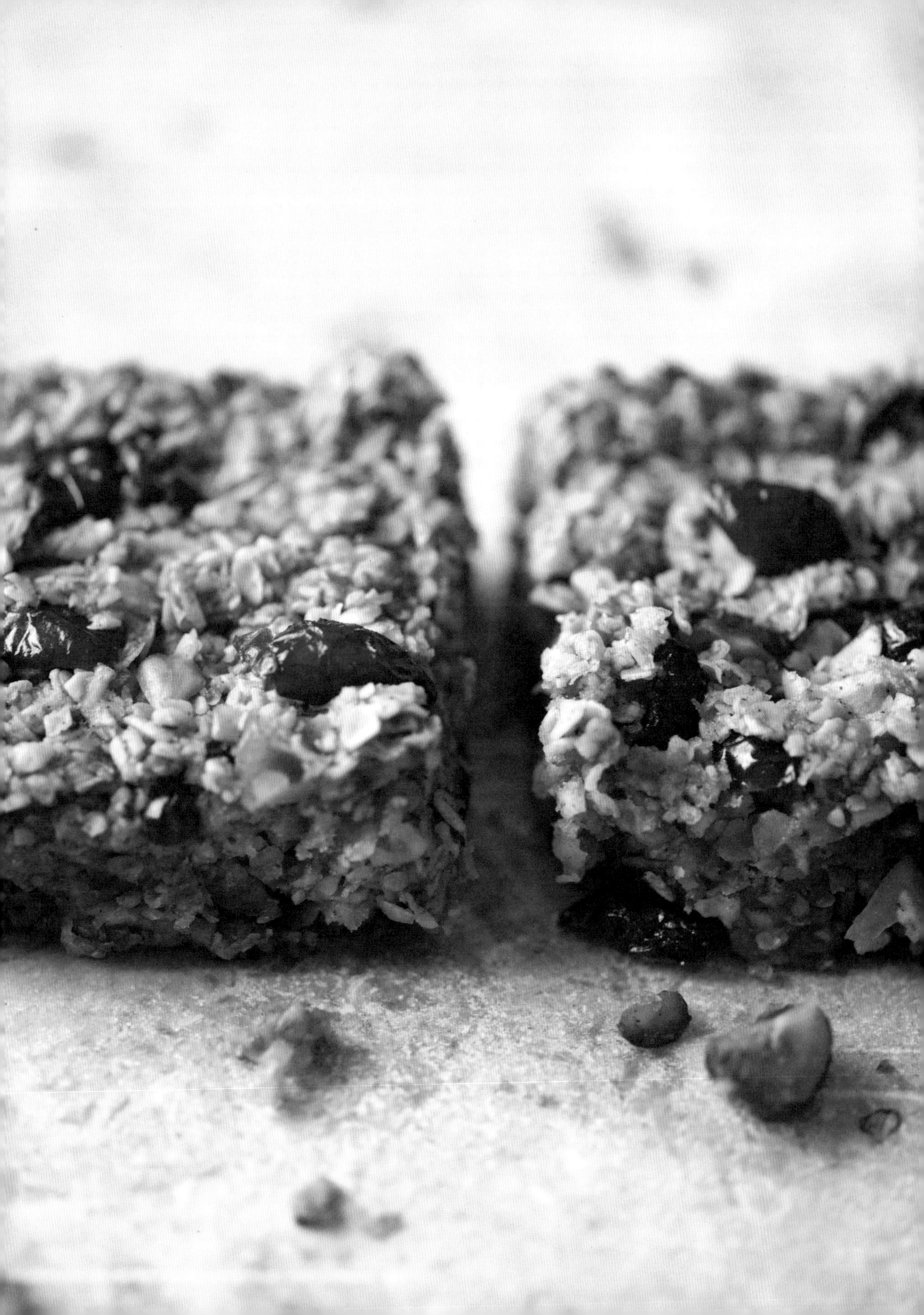

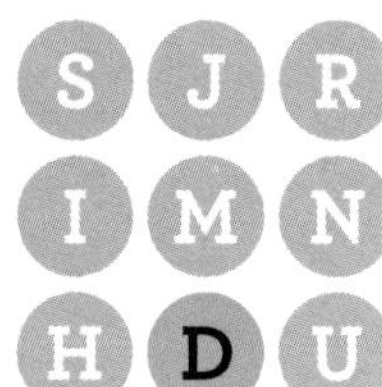

Energy bombs This is an awesome little snack to have in the refrigerator when you need something to nibble on for a boost of energy. Spirulina, a type of algae, is packed with protein, essential fatty acids, and B vitamins. It's easy to find in health food stores.

SERVES 10 TO 12

2 cups pitted dates
2½ cups raw walnuts
3 teaspoons spirulina powder
dry unsweetened coconut, to coat

Put the dates, walnuts, and spirulina into a food processor, and process at full speed until a stiff paste forms.

Sprinkle the dry unsweetened coconut on a plate and have another clean plate handy. Processing the ingredients at high speed will have squeezed the oil from the walnuts, so the paste will be very oily. Break off thumb-size pieces of paste, roll them into balls, then roll in the dry unsweetened coconut. Place the coated balls on a clean plate.

Once all the paste has been rolled into balls, place in the refrigerator for several hours, which will make them firmer and give them a fantastic chewy texture.

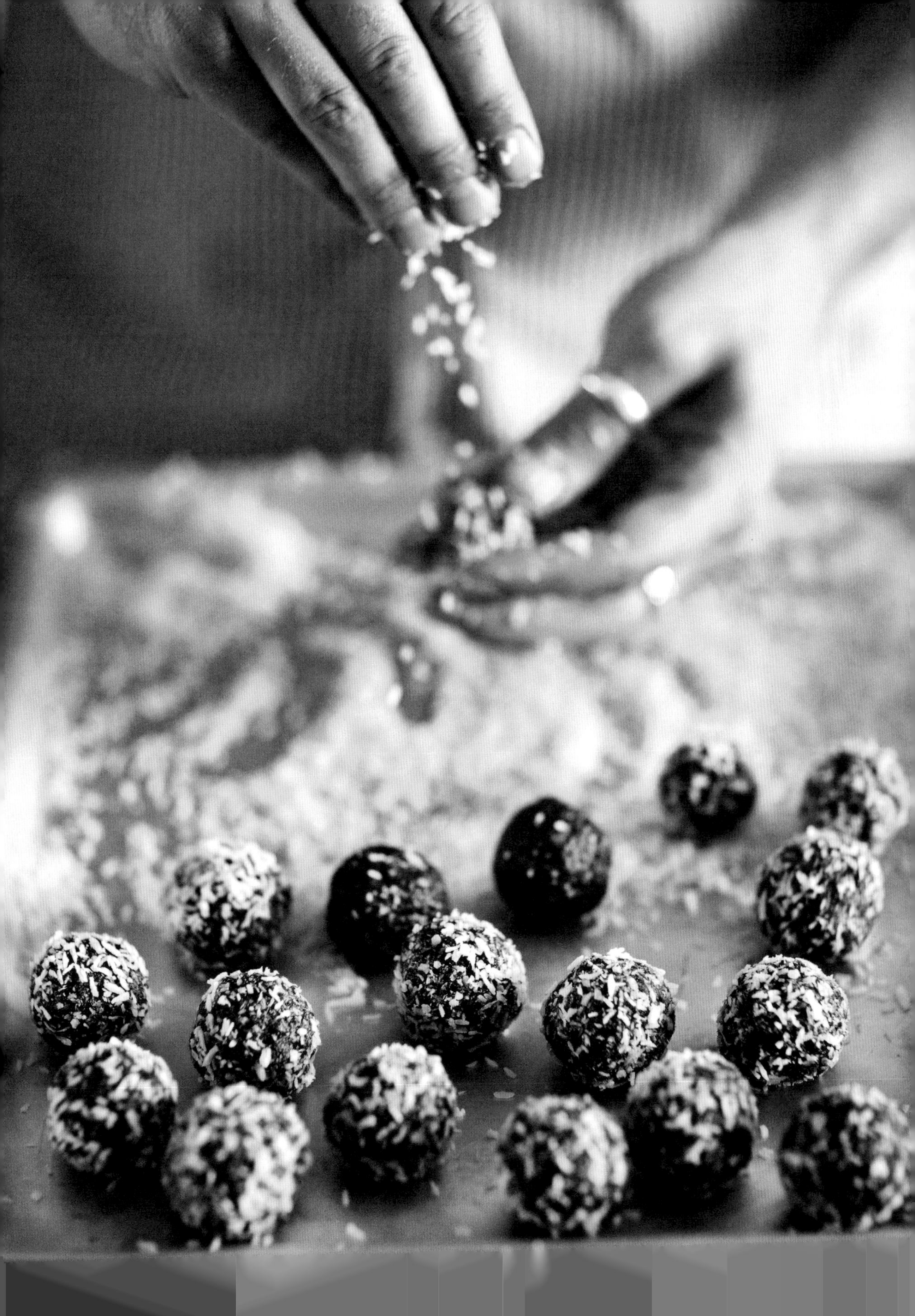

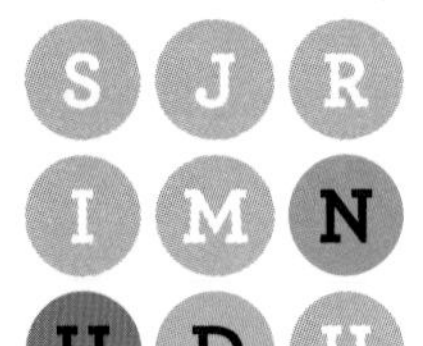

MENTAL HEALTH & NERVOUS SYSTEM *Insomnia, Stress*
HEART & CIRCULATION *High cholesterol*
DIGESTIVE SYSTEM *Constipation*

Banana-peanut oat bars

These gorgeous treats have a wonderful, cakey feel to them, and it's hard to believe that they're actually good for you. I've used coconut oil in this recipe; it's a far healthier baking fat than butter, and is really easy to buy now. Most grocery stores or health food stores will have it.

MAKES 8 BARS

- 1 tablespoon coconut oil, plus extra for greasing
- 3 very ripe bananas
- 1 tablespoon honey
- 2 tablespoons crunchy peanut butter
- generous 2 cups rolled oats
- 2 tablespoons flax seeds

Preheat the oven to 350°F and grease an 8-inch square baking pan with a little coconut oil.

In a bowl, mash the bananas with a fork until almost smooth. Next, melt the coconut oil, honey, and peanut butter together over low heat in a large pan. Once melted, remove from the heat and stir in the mashed bananas.

Once the bananas are thoroughly mixed in, stir in the oats and flax seeds and mix well until a sticky mixture is formed.

Transfer this mixture to the prepared pan, pressing down well to ensure the mixture is compact, then bake in the oven for 20 minutes, or until golden brown.

Let cool completely before cutting into pieces.

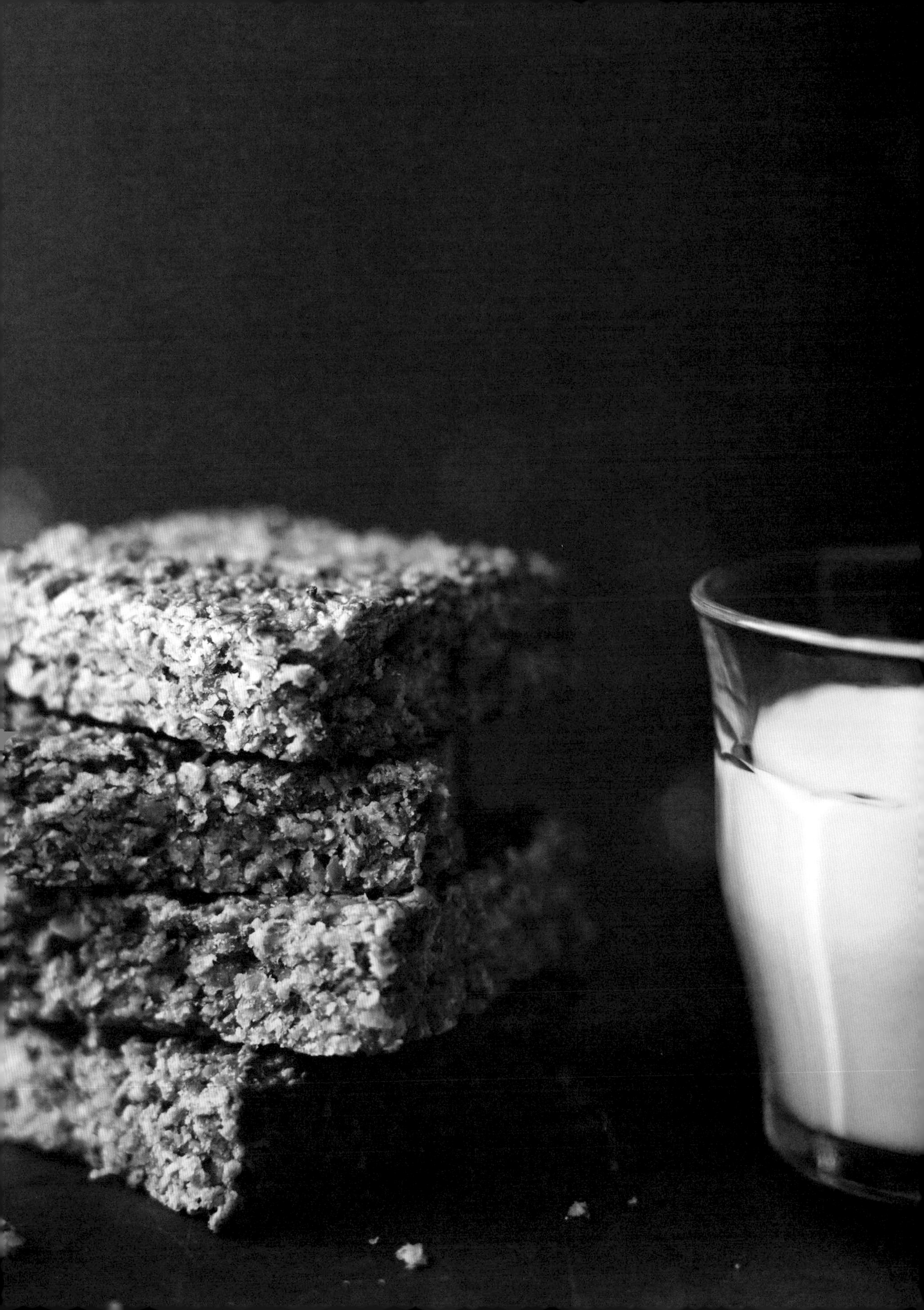

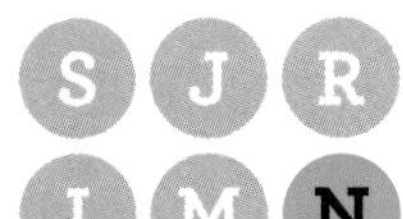

MENTAL HEALTH & NERVOUS SYSTEM *Depression, Stress*
HEART & CIRCULATION *High blood pressure, High cholesterol*
DIGESTIVE SYSTEM *Constipation*

Fabulous refrigerator cakes

Refrigerator cakes are a cinch to make. They are sweet, delicious, and so dense in nutrients that one of these will keep you going for hours. It's always a pleasure when good, wholesome, healthy food tastes so naughty. Get stuck in!

MAKES 8 PIECES

½ cup mixed seeds (such as flax, pumpkin, sesame, and sunflower)
3 handfuls goji berries
handful pitted dates
4 tablespoons cacao powder
1 teaspoon dry unsweetened coconut
1 teaspoon ground cinnamon
4 tablespoons coconut oil
1 tablespoon nuts, such as pecans, walnuts, or brazil nuts, chopped
1 tablespoon dried fruit, such as dried apricots or cranberries, chopped

Place all the ingredients except the coconut oil, nuts, and dried fruit in a food processor, setting aside about 1 tablespoon of the seeds and goji berries, and pulse a few times to start creating a stiff, coarse mixture.

Place the coconut oil in a heatproof bowl, then sit the bowl in some freshly boiled water. The oil will melt in a matter of seconds. Add the melted oil to the rest of the ingredients in the food processor. Process the ingredients at full speed until they have combined thoroughly into a firm paste.

Line an 8-inch square baking pan with baking parchment, turn the mixture into the pan, and press down firmly to completely fill it. Sprinkle the reserved seeds and goji berries over the top, along with the chopped nuts and fruit, and press down lightly. Place in the refrigerator for 3 hours, or until firm. Slice into 8 even pieces.

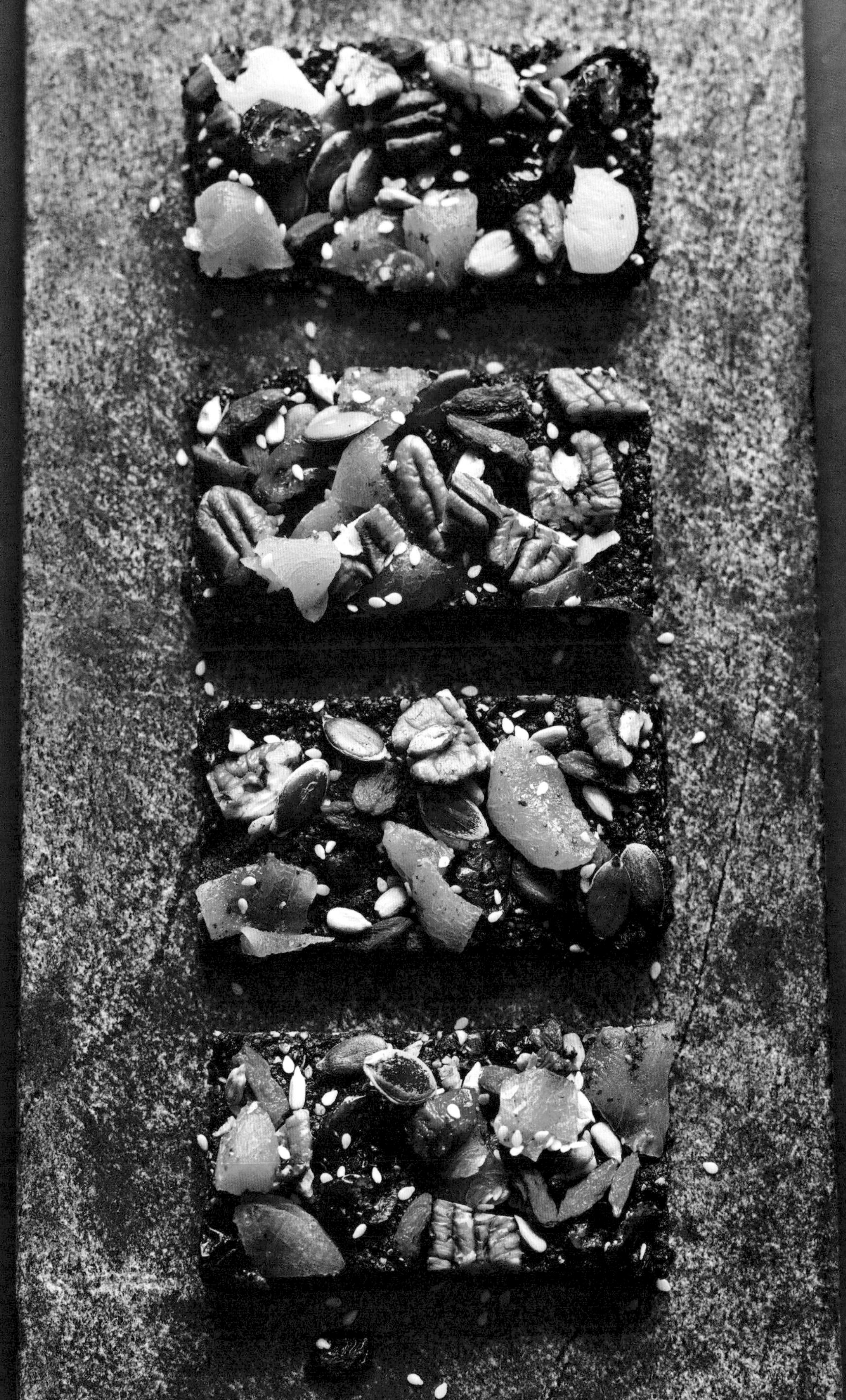

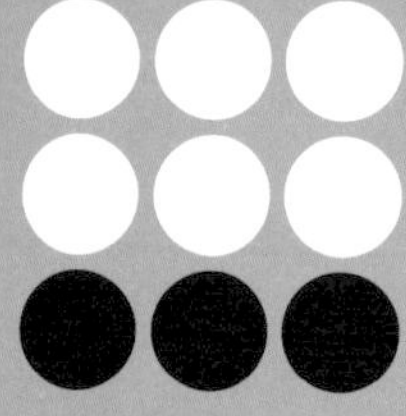

Quick main courses

These recipes make perfect, speedy weekday evening meals. They're tasty, satisfying, and full of nutrients, as well as being pretty easy to whip up in a matter of minutes, so they're perfect after a long day at work.

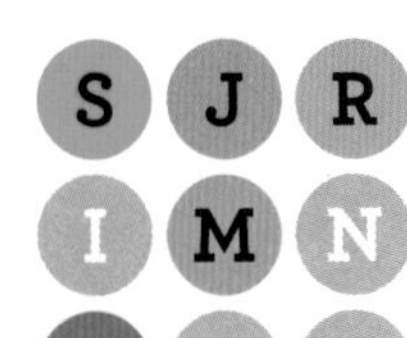

SKIN *Acne*
JOINTS & BONES *Bursitis*
RESPIRATORY SYSTEM *Asthma*
METABOLIC SYSTEM *Diabetes (Type 2)*
HEART & CIRCULATION *High blood pressure, High cholesterol*

Omega pesto pasta This is a delicious and incredibly filling dish, packed with effective phytochemical compounds. Simple, potent, tasty.

SERVES 2

2 cups walnuts
5 loosely packed cups fresh basil leaves (from 2 large bunches)
2 garlic cloves
1 tablespoon ground flax seeds
1 tablespoon grated Parmesan cheese
1 tablespoon extra-virgin olive oil, plus extra for cooking
1 tablespoon flaxseed oil
½ pound whole wheat penne pasta
3 handfuls baby spinach or arugula
sea salt and black pepper

Put the walnuts, basil, garlic, ground flax seeds, Parmesan, olive, and flaxseed oils in a small food processor, and process to make a smooth pesto.

Bring a large pan of salted water to a boil, add the pasta, and cook for 8 to 10 minutes (check the directions on the package), or until tender but still firm to the bite.

Meanwhile, heat a little olive oil in a large, shallow pan, add the spinach, if using, and cook for 1 to 2 minutes, or until wilted, stirring frequently. Drain the pasta and stir it into the spinach, making sure they are well combined. If using arugula, just stir the arugula leaves through the hot pasta without cooking them first. Season with salt and pepper.

Remove from the heat and stir in the pesto, then serve immediately. It's important that the pesto isn't cooked so as to preserve the delicate but essential fatty acids it contains.

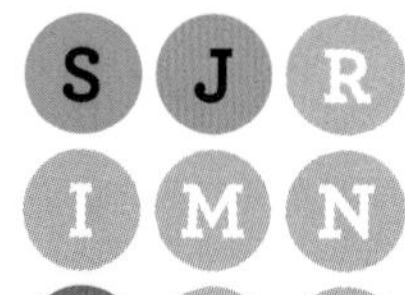

SKIN *Acne, Eczema*
JOINTS & BONES *Arthritis, Bursitis*
HEART & CIRCULATION *High blood pressure, High cholesterol*

Sweet potato and spinach curry

The thought of making a curry from scratch probably scares many of us, but it's really easy once you get into it and understand the flavor combinations of the different spices. That's got to be a winner!

SERVES 3 TO 4

1 tablespoon olive oil
2 red onions, thinly sliced
2 large garlic cloves, minced
1 teaspoon freshly grated ginger
2 green chili peppers, thinly sliced
1 teaspoon ground coriander
1 teaspoon ground cumin
1 teaspoon black mustard seeds
1 heaping teaspoon turmeric
1¾ pounds sweet potatoes, diced into 1¼-inches chunks, skins left on
generous 1½ cups vegetable stock
5 ounces spinach, coarsely chopped
sea salt
large handful fresh cilantro leaves, coarsely torn
1 tablespoon toasted slivered almonds

Heat the olive oil in a large pan over medium heat, add the onions, garlic, ginger, and chili peppers, and cook for 4 to 5 minutes, or until softened. Add all the spices and stir until they become fragrant, about 30 seconds.

Add the sweet potatoes and stock and simmer for 15 to 20 minutes, or until the sweet potatoes are soft.

Next, add the spinach and season with salt. Once the spinach has wilted, sprinkle with the cilantro and slivered almonds and serve immediately.

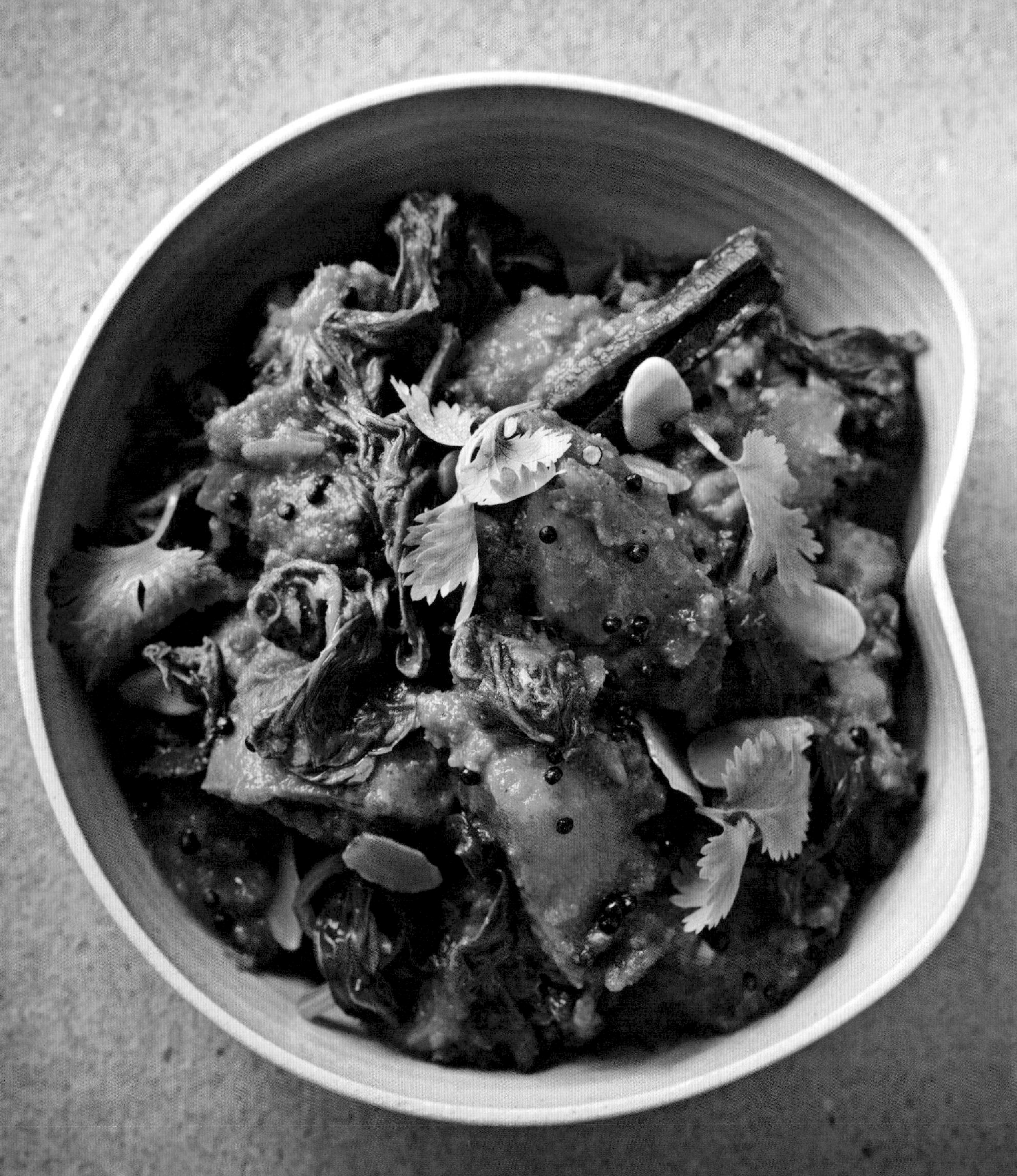

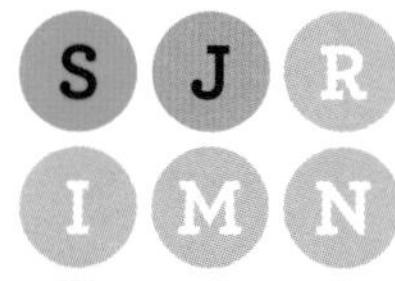

SKIN *Eczema, Psoriasis*
JOINTS & BONES *Rickets*
HEART & CIRCULATION *High blood pressure, Heart disease*
DIGESTIVE SYSTEM *Bloating*

Red bell peppers stuffed with herbed goat cheese

A fabulous infusion of flavors. Culinary herbs deliver masses of pharmacological activity, and this lovely dish is jam-packed with them.

SERVES 2

2 red bell peppers
scant 1 cup soft goat cheese
handful fresh parsley leaves, minced
handful fresh cilantro leaves, minced
handful fresh dill, minced
1 teaspoon olive oil
2 teaspoons lemon juice
sea salt and black pepper
1 teaspoon pine nuts

Preheat the oven to 400°F. Cut the bell peppers in half lengthwise and scrape out the seeds and white membranes. Place the pepper halves cut-side down on a baking pan and add a little water. Bake in the oven for about 15 minutes, or until tender.

Meanwhile, place the goat cheese in a bowl and break it up with a fork. Stir the herbs into the goat cheese along with the olive oil and lemon juice, and season with salt and pepper. Mix well to create a lovely, smooth herbed cheese.

Remove the peppers from the oven, turn them over to expose the insides, and fill the halves with the cheese mixture. Top with the pine nuts. Return to the oven for another 10 to 12 minutes, or until lightly browned, then remove and serve with a salad.

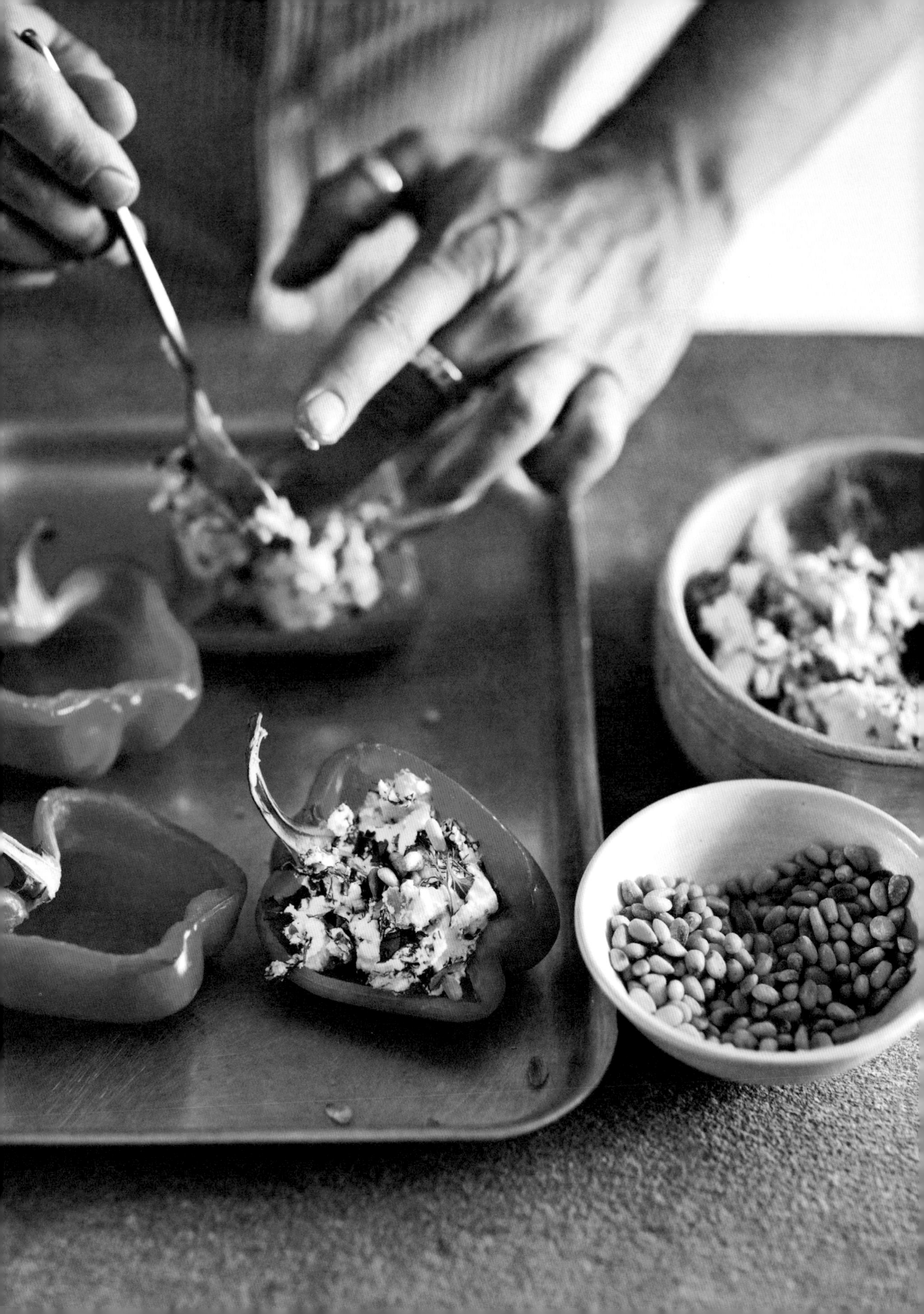

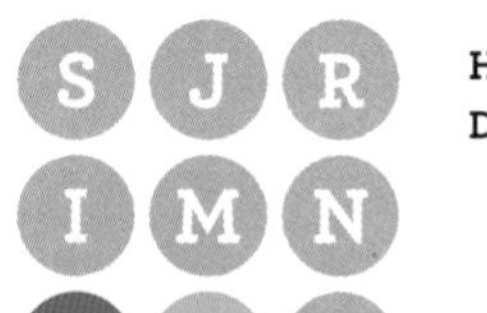

HEART & CIRCULATION *Heart disease*
DIGESTIVE SYSTEM *Constipation*

Zucchini stuffed with balsamic onions and goat cheese This is a lovely, light dish, full of flavor and nutritional value.

SERVES 1
olive oil, for cooking
½ red onion, finely sliced
1 teaspoon balsamic vinegar
1 teaspoon honey
1 large zucchini
sea salt and black pepper
generous ¼ cup soft goat cheese

Heat a little olive oil in a small pan and add the red onion. Cook for 4 to 5 minutes, or until softened, then add the balsamic vinegar and honey. Stir well and keep cooking until the mixture becomes sticky. Set aside.

Meanwhile, preheat the oven to 400°F. Cut the zucchini in half lengthwise. Scoop out the seeds with a teaspoon to create a trough. Place the zucchini, trough facing downward, on a baking sheet or roasting pan with a small amount of water in the bottom. Bake in the oven for about 15 minutes, or until the zucchini begins to soften.

At this stage, carefully drain any remaining water out of the pan. Turn the zucchini halves over and fill the troughs with the onion mixture. Season with salt and pepper. Crumble the goat cheese over the top, and return to the oven for another 5 to 8 minutes, or until the cheese is lightly golden. Serve immediately.

S J R
I M N
H D U

SKIN *Acne, Eczema*
HEART & CIRCULATION *Heart disease*

Antioxidant salad with orange mustard dressing

I'm not overly keen on the term "superfood" and the hype that goes with it, but there are a couple of ingredients in this dish that have certainly come under that label in the past. They're great because they are antioxidant and rich in vitamins, but they won't make you fly or walk on water any time soon.

SERVES 2

- ¼ butternut squash, unpeeled, chopped into small cubes
- olive oil, for drizzling
- 2 cups broccoli florets
- 2½ cups baby spinach
- 1 cup cherry tomatoes
- seeds of 1 pomegranate
- sea salt and black pepper
- juice of 1 orange
- 1 heaping teaspoon whole grain mustard
- 1 tablespoon olive oil

Preheat the oven to 400°F. Place the butternut squash in a roasting pan and drizzle with olive oil. Roast for 20 minutes, or until softened and the skin is starting to caramelize.

While the squash is cooking, bring a pan of water to boil, add the broccoli, and cook for 3 to 4 minutes, or just long enough for it to start to soften and turn bright green.

Place the spinach and cherry tomatoes in a salad bowl. Add the cooked squash and broccoli and the pomegranate seeds, season with salt and pepper, and toss well.

Combine the orange juice, mustard, and olive oil in a bowl, and mix thoroughly. Dress the salad and toss again.

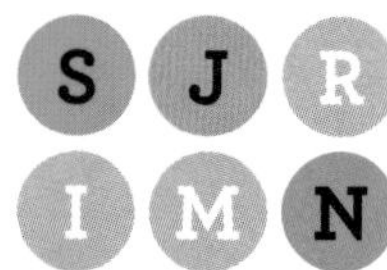

SKIN *Eczema, Psoriasis*
JOINTS & BONES *Bursitis*
MENTAL HEALTH & NERVOUS SYSTEM *Anxiety*
HEART & CIRCULATION *High cholesterol*
DIGESTIVE SYSTEM *Bloating, Crohn's disease*

Baked sweet potatoes with omega hummus

This is a lovely, filling dish that's packed with soluble fiber and the phytonutrients beta-sitosterol, beta-carotene, and omega-3 fatty acids.

SERVES 2

2 medium sweet potatoes
1 14-ounce can chickpeas, drained
1 tablespoon sesame seeds
2 tablespoons flaxseed oil
1 garlic clove, minced
juice of ½ lemon
sea salt and black pepper
handful fresh parsley or cilantro leaves, coarsely chopped (optional)

Preheat the oven to 400°F. Put the sweet potatoes on a baking sheet and roast in the oven for 40 minutes, or until very soft when squeezed.

Meanwhile, place the chickpeas, sesame seeds, flaxseed oil, garlic, and lemon juice into a blender or food processor, season with salt and pepper, and process into a smooth hummus.

When the sweet potatoes are cooked, cut each one in half lengthwise and pile a big dollop of the hummus on top of them. Scatter with the herbs, if using. Serve immediately.

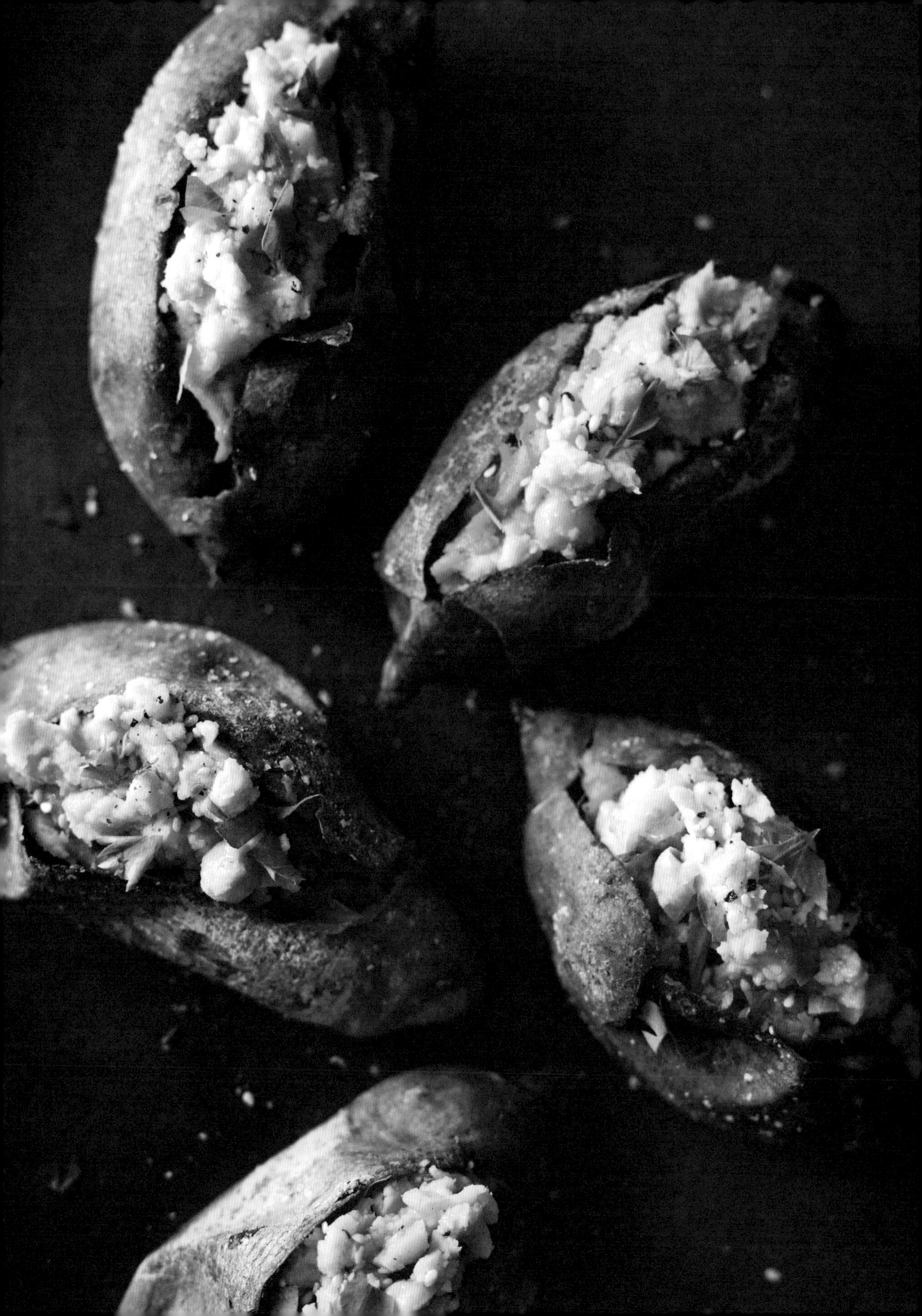

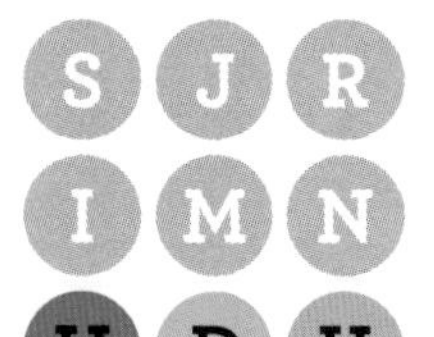

HEART & CIRCULATION *High blood pressure, High cholesterol*
DIGESTIVE SYSTEM *Constipation*
REPRODUCTIVE & URINARY SYSTEMS *Prostate health*

Whole wheat bean quesadillas

I just love bean quesadillas. They remind me of my first job in a health food store in the late 1990s. This store made the best bean quesadillas ever, and I'd treat myself to one at the end of every shift. Gooey, rich, filling: they are comforting in a million ways.

SERVES 2

- olive oil, for cooking and brushing
- 2 garlic cloves, minced
- 1 small green chili pepper, seeded and minced
- ½ teaspoon ground cumin
- 1 14-ounce can mixed beans, drained
- 1 cup fresh cherry tomatoes, coarsely chopped
- sea salt and black pepper
- 2 large or 4 small whole wheat tortillas
- small bunch fresh cilantro, coarsely chopped
- large handful low-fat cheddar cheese, grated

Heat a little olive oil in a pan, add the garlic, chili pepper, and cumin and cook gently for 2 minutes.

Add the beans and the tomatoes, and continue to cook for 10 to 15 minutes, or until the liquid from the tomatoes has virtually vanished, and you are left with a thick tomato-bean stew. Season it with salt and pepper. Preheat the oven to 350°F.

Lay the tortillas out flat, spoon some of the mixture on the side of each one, then pat it down gently. Sprinkle some cilantro over the top of the beans, then half the grated cheddar on top of that. Fold the tortilla in half to make a parcel.

Place the folded quesadillas on a baking sheet. Bake in the oven for about 10 minutes, or until golden. Alternatively, brush a grill pan with a little olive oil and place over medium-high heat. Toast the quesadillas on each side for 4–6 minutes. Serve immediately.

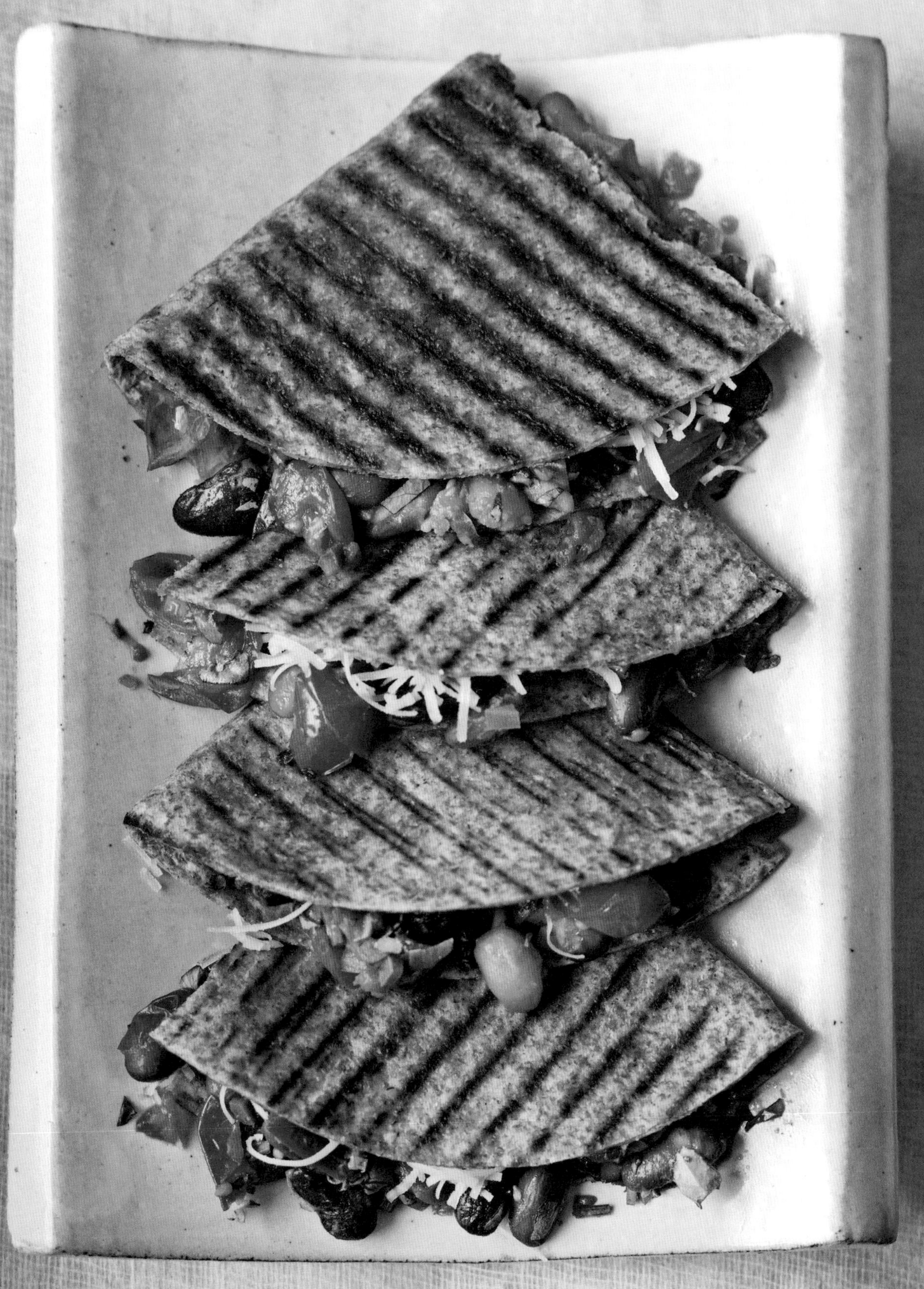

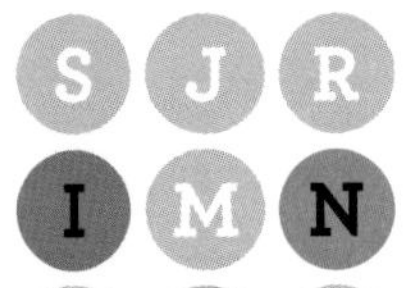

IMMUNE SYSTEM *Colds & flu*
MENTAL HEALTH & NERVOUS SYSTEM
Anxiety, Insomnia, Migraine, Stress
DIGESTIVE SYSTEM *Constipation*

Kale and potato salad with peanut chili sauce

You may think raw kale will be tough, chewy, and not exactly a treat. But this is a wonderful way to give it the same texture as cooked kale, without damaging the nutrients.

SERVES 2

8 new potatoes
1 small bunch raw curly kale
1–2 tablespoons olive oil
sea salt
2 garlic cloves, minced
1 red chili pepper, minced
3 heaping tablespoons good-quality peanut butter (no added salt or sugar)
1 tablespoon dark soy sauce
2 teaspoons honey
½ teaspoon Chinese five-spice powder
10 cherry tomatoes, halved
small handful fresh cilantro leaves

Put the new potatoes in a pan, cover with boiling water, and simmer for 15 to 20 minutes, or until tender. Drain well and set aside.

Put the kale in a large bowl and tear the leaves into small bite-size pieces, discarding any thick, tough stems. Drizzle the olive oil and a good pinch of salt over the kale and massage it in with both hands. This will make it wilt and take on the same texture as cooked kale. Once soft and wilted, move on to making the sauce.

Put the minced garlic and chili pepper, peanut butter, soy sauce, honey, five-spice powder, and 4 tablespoons water in a small bowl, and mix well. The mixture will look as though it has separated at first, but keep stirring and it will come together to make a wonderful satay-like sauce. If it is too thick, add a little more water.

Add the sauce to the kale and stir well. Once all of the sauce is mixed into the kale, cut the potatoes and cherry tomatoes in half, and add them to the kale and stir again. Garnish with cilantro and serve.

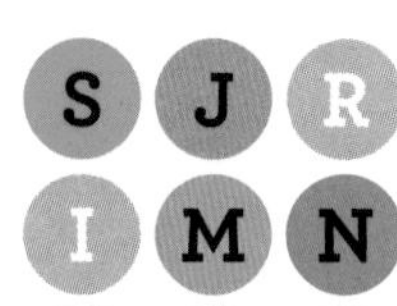

SKIN *Acne, Eczema, Psoriasis*
JOINTS & BONES *Rickets*
METABOLIC SYSTEM *Diabetes (Type 2)*
MENTAL HEALTH & NERVOUS SYSTEM *Anxiety, Stress*
REPRODUCTIVE & URINARY SYSTEMS *Problematic periods*

Smoked trout and quinoa salad

This is a lovely salad that makes a great light lunch or dinner. Don't be put off by quinoa—it's a very easy and versatile ingredient to use, and extremely good for you.

SERVES 2

scant 1 cup quinoa
1 teaspoon vegetable stock powder or 1 vegetable stock cube
2 smoked trout fillets (about 3 ounces each)
small bunch fresh parsley leaves, minced
1 red bell pepper, finely diced
1 tablespoon capers
sea salt and black pepper
2 tablespoons olive oil
2 teaspoons balsamic vinegar
½ teaspoon dried mixed herbs
2 handfuls fresh arugula leaves

Put the quinoa in a pan, cover with freshly boiled water, and add the vegetable stock. Simmer for 10 to 15 minutes, or until just tender. Drain well.

Break up the trout fillets into bite-size pieces.

Place the cooked quinoa in a salad bowl, add the flaked trout, parsley, diced pepper, and capers and stir well. Season with salt and pepper.

Combine the olive oil, balsamic vinegar, and mixed herbs together to make a dressing, and drizzle it over the salad. Top with fresh arugula and serve.

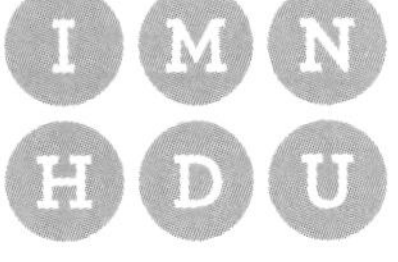

SKIN *Acne, Eczema, Psoriasis*
RESPIRATORY SYSTEM *Asthma*

Roasted bell peppers with white bean mash

There's something about white bean mash that I love—it's so creamy and flavorful. This dish is seriously nutrient-packed, and couldn't be easier to make.

SERVES 4

- 4 bell peppers (I prefer to use 2 different colors for contrast), cut into long, wide strips
- 2 zucchini, cut into 1-inch chunks
- extra-virgin olive oil, for cooking and mashing
- 2 garlic cloves, crushed
- sea salt and black pepper
- 1 14-ounce can cannellini beans, drained
- 1 14-ounce can lima beans, drained
- small handful fresh cilantro leaves, coarsely chopped
- juice of ½ lemon
- mixed salad greens, to serve

Preheat the oven to 350°F. Put the peppers and zucchini in a roasting pan, drizzle with olive oil, season with salt and pepper, and add half the crushed garlic. Stir well. Roast in the oven for 15 to 20 minutes, or until soft.

Meanwhile, heat a little olive oil in a pan, add the remaining garlic, and cook gently for 1 to 2 minutes, until it begins to turn fragrant. Add the drained beans and stir well.

Mash the bean mixture in the same way you would mash potatoes, using a handheld masher. Instead of adding milk and butter like in a traditional mash, add a little extra-virgin olive oil to give it a creamy texture.

Stir in the chopped cilantro and the lemon juice, and season with salt and pepper. Serve the roasted vegetables and bean mash with a mixed green salad.

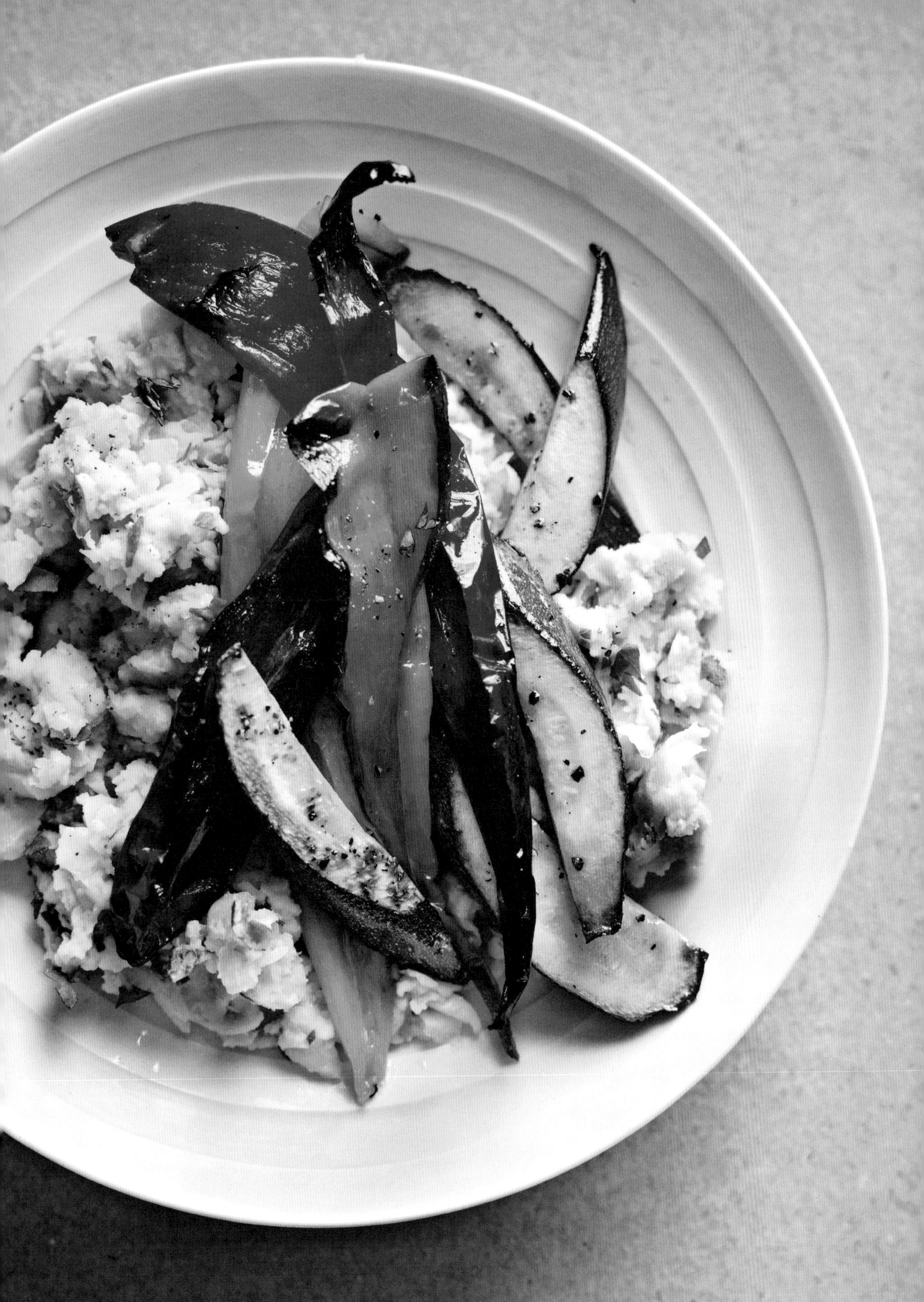

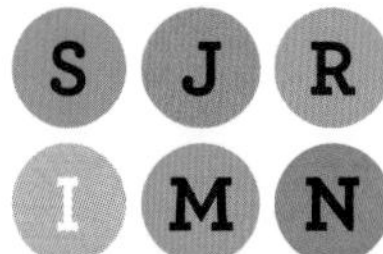
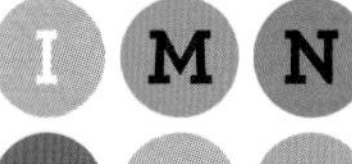
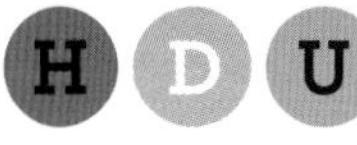

SKIN *Acne, Eczema*
JOINTS & BONES *Arthritis, Bursitis*
RESPIRATORY SYSTEM *Asthma*
METABOLIC SYSTEM *Diabetes (Type 2)*
MENTAL HEALTH & NERVOUS SYSTEM *Depression*
HEART & CIRCULATION *High cholesterol*
REPRODUCTIVE & URINARY SYSTEMS *Polycystic ovary syndrome*

Tuna steaks with sweet potato wedges and greens

This is a healthy take on fish and chips—well, it is to me at least! It contains some very nutritious ingredients, and it's fabulous for the health of many body systems.

SERVES 2

- 2 large sweet potatoes
- olive oil, for drizzling and cooking
- 4 ounces greens, such as Swiss chard, kale, or bok choy, shredded (about 4 cups)
- 2 garlic cloves, minced
- 1 red chili pepper, minced
- 2 tuna steaks, about 5 ounces each
- sea salt and black pepper

Preheat the oven to 350°F. Cut the unpeeled sweet potatoes lengthwise into long, thin wedges. Drizzle the wedges with a little olive oil, season with salt and pepper, and cook in the oven for about 20 minutes, or until they start to brown and the skin begins to crisp. Turn them over at least once, too.

Heat a little olive oil in a pan on a medium heat, add the greens, and fry for 5 to 8 minutes, or until they have turned a much brighter green color. At this stage, add the garlic and chili pepper, season with salt and pepper, and stir well.

Heat a nonstick skillet or griddle with a tiny amount of olive oil on a medium heat Add the tuna and sear it for 3 to 4 minutes on each side. If the thought of the middle of the tuna being pink really puts you off, you can of course cook it for longer, but cooking it lightly does preserve more of that vital omega 3. Slice the tuna and arrange it on top of the greens, then serve immediately.

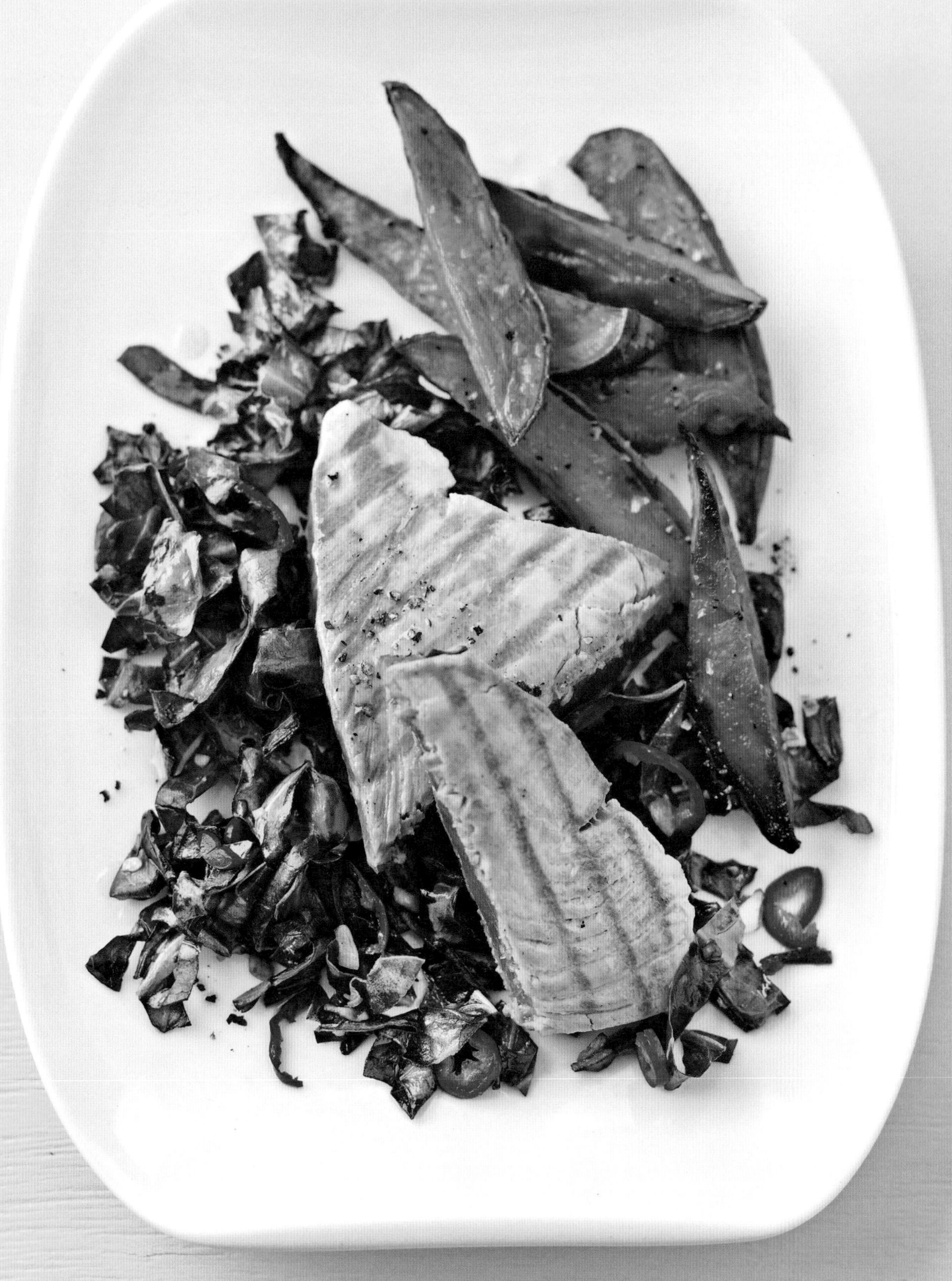

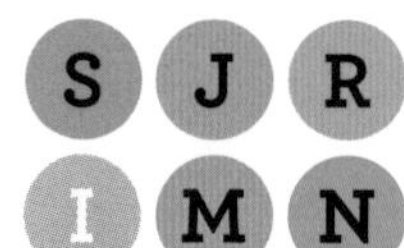

SKIN *Acne*
JOINTS & BONES *Arthritis, Osteoporosis*
RESPIRATORY SYSTEM *Asthma*
METABOLIC SYSTEM *Diabetes (Type 2)*
MENTAL HEALTH & NERVOUS SYSTEM *Anxiety, Depression*
HEART & CIRCULATION *High blood pressure, High cholesterol*
REPRODUCTIVE & URINARY SYSTEMS *Endometriosis*

Sesame soy salmon and vegetables with coconut rice

This is a lovely, filling dish with a wonderful Asian-fusion vibe. It's guaranteed to be a dinner party favorite, too.

SERVES 2

2 tablespoons low-salt soy sauce
1 teaspoon sesame oil
1 teaspoon honey
2 large salmon fillets, about 5 ounces each
¾ cup brown rice
1 14-ounce can coconut milk
2 tablespoons dry unsweetened coconut
olive oil, for cooking
1 garlic clove, minced
1 large red onion, thinly sliced
1 small carrot, cut into thin strips
½ zucchini, cut into thin strips
handful baby spinach
sea salt

Mix together 1 tablespoon soy sauce with the sesame oil and honey, and stir well to create a marinade. Pour over the salmon and let marinate for at least an hour, or overnight.

Put the rice in a pan and cover with salted boiling water. Simmer over medium heat until half cooked, about 10 minutes (check the directions on the package). Add the coconut milk and continue to simmer until the rice is soft and tender. You may need to add a little extra water. Add the coconut and stir well. Transfer to a warmed dish and set aside.

Heat a nonstick skillet over medium heat, add the salmon and its marinade, and cook for 6 to 8 minutes, turning once.

Meanwhile, heat a little olive oil in a large pan or wok and add the garlic, onion, carrot, and zucchini. Stir-fry for 2 to 3 minutes, until soft. Add the spinach and remaining soy sauce, and cook for 1 minute. Once the salmon and vegetables are cooked, serve immediately with the coconut rice.

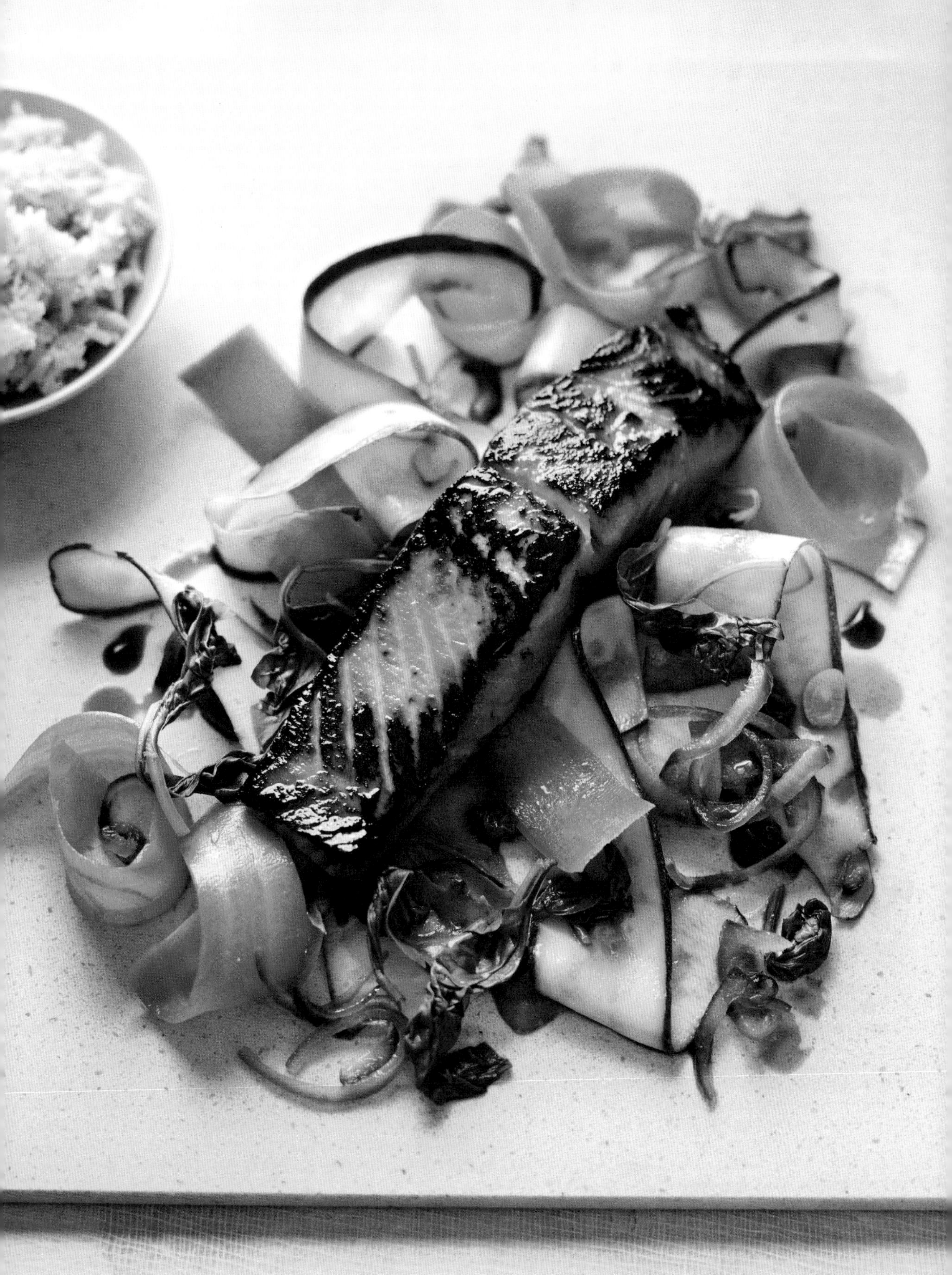

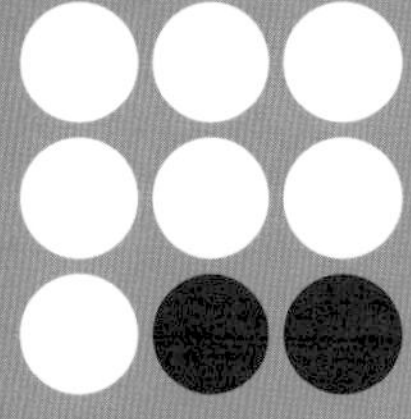

Weekend main courses

These dishes are ideal for when you have a bit more time on your hands to create something special. They involve a few more steps than the quick main courses, but they're worth the effort, and many of them are great dinner party dishes.

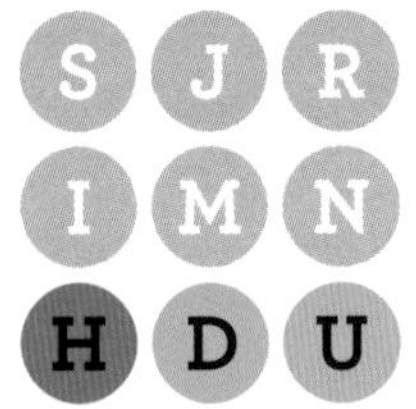

HEART & CIRCULATION *High cholesterol*
DIGESTIVE SYSTEM *Bloating, Constipation, IBS*
REPRODUCTIVE & URINARY SYSTEMS *Prostate health*

Vegetable crumble with cheesy oat topping

This is serious comfort food. It's full of antioxidants, potent phytochemical compounds, fiber, and, most important of all, flavor.

SERVES 3 TO 4

olive oil, for cooking
1 large red onion, minced
2 garlic cloves, minced
1 large zucchini, chopped
1 small eggplant, diced
2 red bell peppers, diced
scant 2 cups strained tomatoes
sea salt and black pepper

For the topping:
generous 1 cup rolled oats
scant ⅓ cup whole wheat flour
2 tablespoons grated Parmesan cheese
3 tablespoons olive oil

Heat a little olive oil in a pan, add the onion and garlic and cook gently for 4 to 5 minutes, or until softened.

Add the chopped zucchini, eggplant, and peppers and continue cooking until the vegetables start to soften. Preheat the oven to 400°F.

Add the strained tomatoes, bring to a simmer, and continue to cook for about another 15 minutes. By this time, the strained tomatoes should have reduced down and the mixture should resemble a thick ratatouille. Season with salt and pepper and transfer to a baking dish.

Meanwhile, make the topping: Mix the oats, flour, and Parmesan together, and then stir in the olive oil, adding just enough to create a bread crumb-like texture.

Sprinkle the topping over the vegetable mixture, and bake for 15 to 20 minutes, or until golden brown. Let stand for a few minutes before serving.

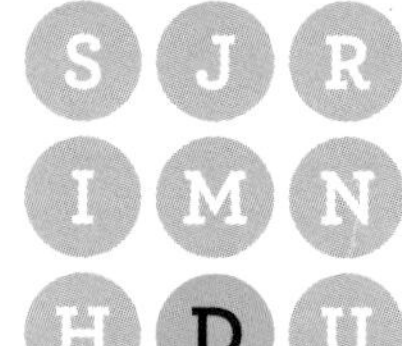

Red beet and pea risotto with mint and feta

Beets and mint may sound a bit like chalk and cheese, but trust me, it really works! The freshness of the mint brings the earthy red beets to life. The medicinal properties of this dish are outstanding, too.

SERVES 2 TO 3

olive oil, for cooking
1 large red onion, minced
2 garlic cloves, minced
generous 1 cup arborio rice
3 medium cooked red beets, cubed
4 cups vegetable stock (made from a stock cube or bouillon powder)
sea salt and black pepper
1¾ cups frozen peas
handful fresh mint, minced
¾ cup crumbled feta cheese

Heat a little olive oil in a pan, add the onion and garlic, and cook for 4 to 5 minutes, or until the onion is soft. Add the rice and cook for another minute. Add two of the beets, setting aside one for later.

Add the vegetable stock little by little, until the rice is soft and just tender, stirring frequently (this can take up to 30 minutes). It should be fairly moist, but not too liquid. Season with salt and pepper.

When the rice is almost cooked, add the peas and mint and cook for another 2 to 3 minutes.

Place the remaining beets in a small food processor and process to a coarse purée. Add the purée to the finished risotto, stir well, and serve on warmed plates. Sprinkle some feta over each one.

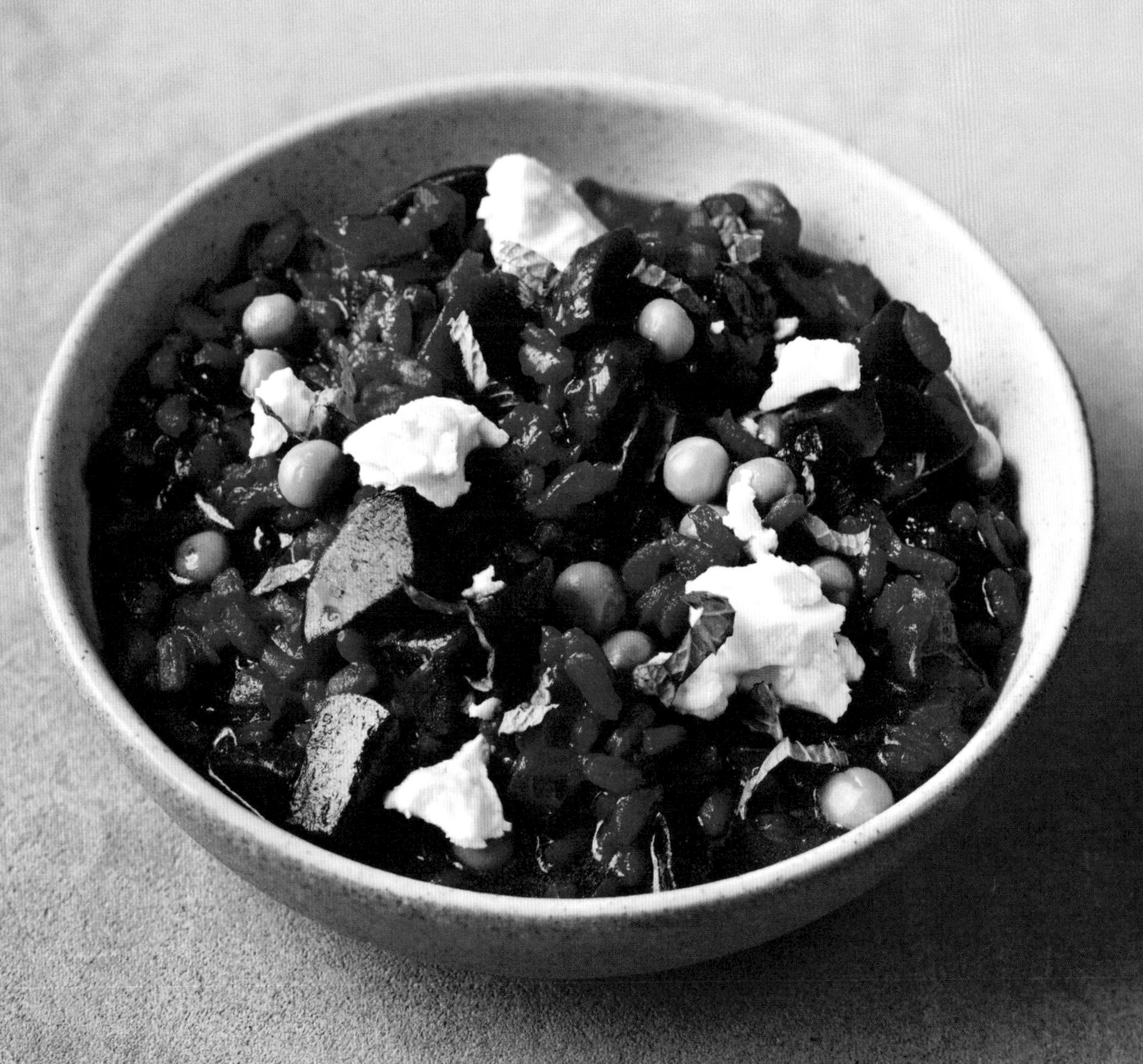

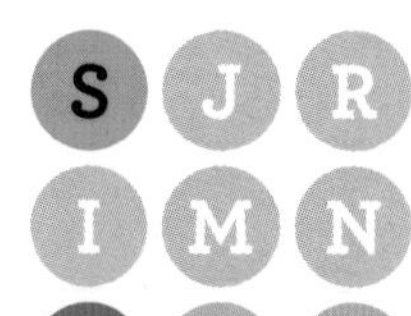

SKIN *Eczema, Psoriasis*
HEART & CIRCULATION *High cholesterol*
DIGESTIVE SYSTEM *Bloating, Constipation*
REPRODUCTIVE & URINARY SYSTEMS
Endometriosis, Polycystic ovary syndrome, Problematic periods

Chickpea and sweet potato beta bake

This recipe is one of my winter favorites. It's just so satisfying on many levels. It's packed with all manner of phytonutrients: beta-carotene, quercetin, inulin, sulfur, phytoestrogens, zinc—you name it.

SERVES 3

2 large sweet potatoes, cut into large chunks, skin on
sea salt and black pepper
olive oil, for cooking
1 red onion, minced
1 garlic clove, minced
2 handfuls baby spinach
1 14-ounce can chickpeas, drained
4 tablespoons sundried tomato paste
Danish blue cheese, to taste (leave it out or substitute with other cheeses, if preferred)

Put the sweet potatoes in a pan, cover with boiling water, and simmer for 8 to 10 minutes, or until soft. Drain well, season with salt and pepper, and mash into a smooth orange purée.

Preheat the oven to 400°F. Heat a little olive oil in a pan and add the red onion and garlic. Cook for 4 to 5 minutes, or until softened. Add the spinach to the onion and garlic and cook for a few minutes more, until the spinach has wilted. Add the chickpeas. Stir well, then add the sundried tomato paste. Season with salt and pepper.

Transfer the chickpea mixture to a baking dish. Put the sweet potato mash on top of this, as though you were making a shepherds' pie.

Crumble the blue cheese over the top, if using, and bake in the oven for 15 to 20 minutes, or until golden and bubbling. Let stand for a few minutes before serving.

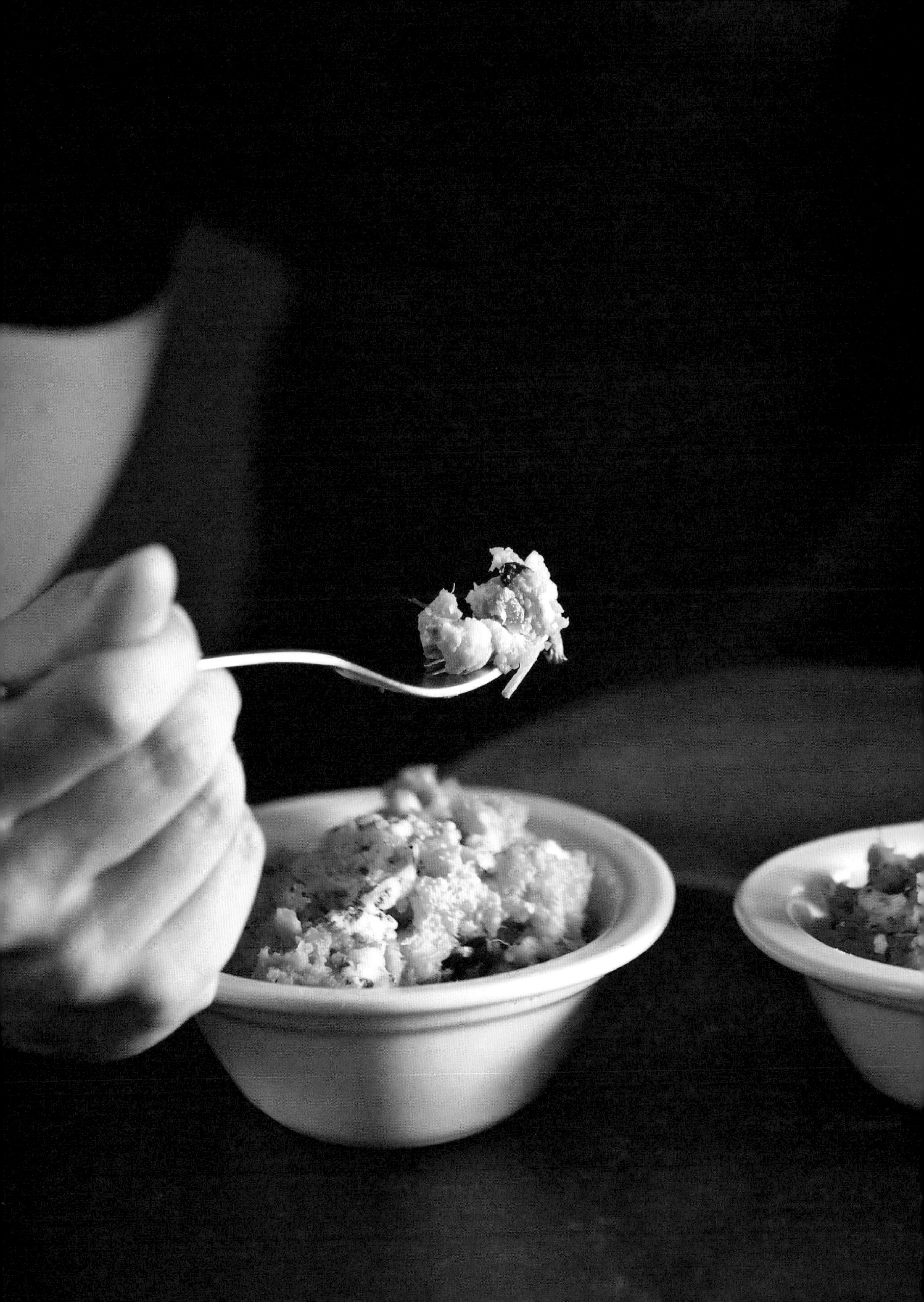

S J R
I M N
H D U

IMMUNE SYSTEM *Colds & flu*
HEART & CIRCULATION *High blood pressure*

Thai green vegetable curry

I love Thai green curry. The powerful chemistry delivered in this dish could fill a book all on its own! Galangal is a powerful relative of ginger. Ordinary fresh ginger will work just fine.

SERVES 3 TO 4

For the curry paste:
2 lemongrass stalks
2 green chili peppers
2 garlic cloves
1 large onion
½-inch piece fresh ginger or galangal, peeled
handful fresh cilantro leaves
4 basil leaves
4 kaffir lime leaves
½ teaspoon white pepper
½ teaspoon ground coriander
3 tablespoons Thai fish sauce or dark soy sauce
1 teaspoon shrimp paste
juice of 1 lime

For the curry:
virgin coconut oil, for frying
1 large zucchini, sliced
½ red pepper, cut into chunks
¼ eggplant, cut into chunks
6–7 pieces baby corn
2 handfuls shiitake mushrooms, sliced
2 handfuls baby spinach
1 14-ounce can coconut milk
¾ cup vegetable stock
1 lime, cut into wedges

Cut the lemon grass, chili peppers, garlic, and onion into large chunks and place in a food processor with the remaining paste ingredients. Process to a pungent, aromatic paste (a word of caution from bitter experience: don't inhale deeply when you take the lid off. You have been warned!).

Heat a little coconut oil in a large pan on a medium heat, add the curry paste, and fry it for a minute or two. It should turn a darker, duller green, and become less pungent.

Add the vegetables, coconut milk, and vegetable stock and simmer for 10 to 15 minutes, or until the vegetables are tender. Serve with lime wedges and cooked brown rice or quinoa.

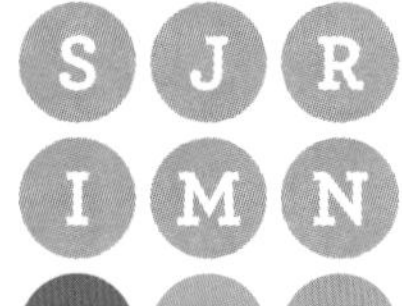

HEART & CIRCULATION *High cholesterol*
DIGESTIVE SYSTEM *Constipation, IBS*
REPRODUCTIVE & URINARY SYSTEMS *Problematic periods*

Baked eggplant with tomato and lentil stuffing Comforting, filling, and flavorful, with a lovely Mediterranean vibe going on.

SERVES 2

1 large eggplant
scant 1 cup red lentils
olive oil, for cooking
½ red onion, minced
2 garlic cloves, minced
sea salt and black pepper
1 red bell pepper, finely chopped
3 tablespoons sundried tomato paste
1 sprig fresh basil, coarsely torn (optional)

Cut the eggplant in half lengthwise and scoop out the flesh, leaving a shell about ¼ inch thick. Chop the scooped-out flesh into ¼-inch pieces.

Preheat the oven to 425°F. Place the hollowed-out eggplant halves face down in a roasting pan, and fill it with water to about ½ inch deep. Bake in the oven for about 15 minutes, or until it begins to soften noticeably.

Place the lentils in a pan, cover with water, and bring to a boil. Reduce the heat and simmer for 15 to 20 minutes, or until they have softened and are beginning to break down.

Heat a little olive oil in a pan, add the onion and garlic, and season with salt and pepper, then cook for 4 to 5 minutes, or until softened. Add the red pepper and eggplant flesh and continue to cook until they have softened. Add the cooked lentils to the onion and garlic, and stir well. Stir in the sundried tomato paste.

Spoon the lentil mixture into the hollowed-out eggplants and return to the oven for 10 to 15 minutes, or until they are nicely roasted and the top of the stuffing is beginning to brown. Scatter with the basil, if using, and serve immediately.

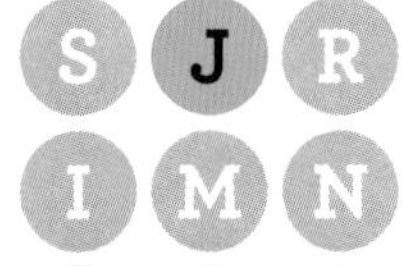

JOINTS & BONES *Rickets*
HEART & CIRCULATION *High blood pressure*
DIGESTIVE SYSTEM *Constipation*

Red beet, red onion, and goat cheese tart

I've got my wonderful mom to thank for this dish. She created a version of it for a family barbecue. One taste and I was hooked! I've rejigged it a bit, but the fundamentals are the same.

SERVES 4 TO 6

olive oil, for cooking
1 large red onion, thinly sliced
1 tablespoon honey
1 sprig fresh thyme leaves
flour, for dusting
1 large sheet ready-made puff pastry
1 egg, lightly beaten
4 large cooked red beets, diced
generous ½ cup crumbled goat cheese (or use feta if you prefer)
generous ⅓ cup pine nuts

Heat a little olive oil in a pan. Add the red onion and cook for 4 to 5 minutes, or until softened. Add the honey and thyme and continue to cook until the onion takes on a caramelized appearance.

Preheat the oven to 400°F. Lightly flour a clean counter and roll out the pastry. Place a large plate on top and cut around it to make a 10-inch diameter circle. With a sharp knife, score another smaller circle about ⅝ inch inside the edge, without cutting all the way through, using a smaller plate as a template if you like. Prick the inner circle with a fork, leaving the rim intact. Brush the rim with beaten egg.

Put the pastry on a baking sheet and bake for 10 to 15 minutes, or until golden. Let cool slightly before pressing down gently on the inner circle to form a rim. Fill the hole with the onions right up to the edge. Sprinkle the diced beets over the onion layer. Finally, sprinkle the cheese over the top, followed by the pine nuts. Return to the oven for about 10 minutes, or until the cheese is golden brown around the edges. Serve immediately—it's great with a green salad.

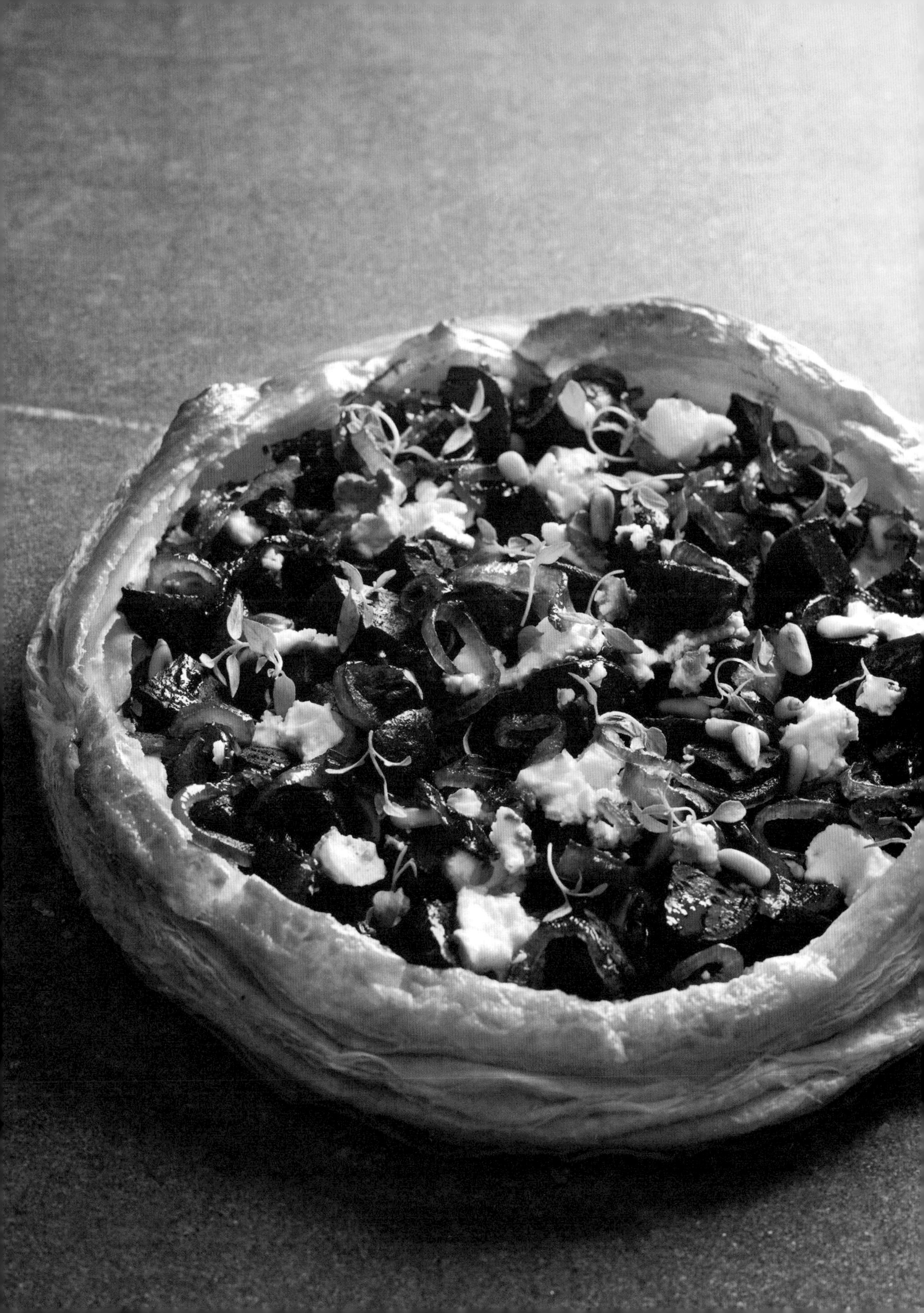

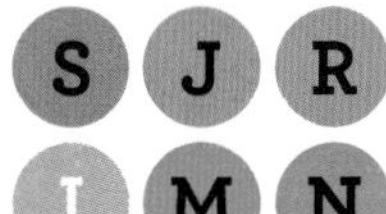
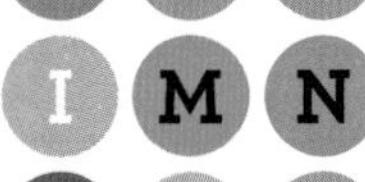
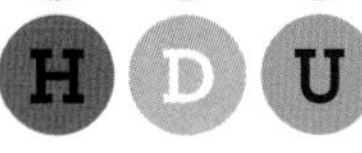

SKIN *Acne, Eczema, Psoriasis*
JOINTS & BONES *Arthritis*
RESPIRATORY SYSTEM *Asthma*
METABOLIC SYSTEM *Diabetes, Type 2*
MENTAL HEATH & NERVOUS SYSTEM *Anxiety, Depression, Stress*
HEART & CIRCULATION *High cholesterol*
REPRODUCTIVE & URINARY SYSTEMS *Menopause, Problematic periods*

Baked salmon with herbed omega crust

This dish is an absolute powerhouse, delivering all the important omega-3 fatty acids, which are vital for virtually every system in the body and provide a whole array of therapeutic benefits.

SERVES 2

- 3 tablespoons ground flax seeds (available in health food stores)
- 1 tablespoon whole grain bread crumbs
- 1 teaspoon dried basil
- 1 teaspoon dried oregano
- 1 teaspoon dried rosemary
- ½ garlic clove, minced
- zest of 1 lemon, plus 1 lemon cut into wedges
- 1 tablespoon olive oil
- sea salt and black pepper
- 2 salmon fillets, about 5 ounces each

Preheat the oven to 375°F and line a baking sheet with aluminum foil. Combine the ground flax seeds, bread crumbs, herbs, garlic, lemon zest, and olive oil in a bowl to make the topping, then season with salt and pepper.

Spread the flax seed mixture over the salmon fillets, flesh side up, and place the fillets on the prepared baking sheet.

Roast in the oven for 8 to 10 minutes, or until the crust is golden brown.

Serve with lemon wedges and a salad of mixed greens.

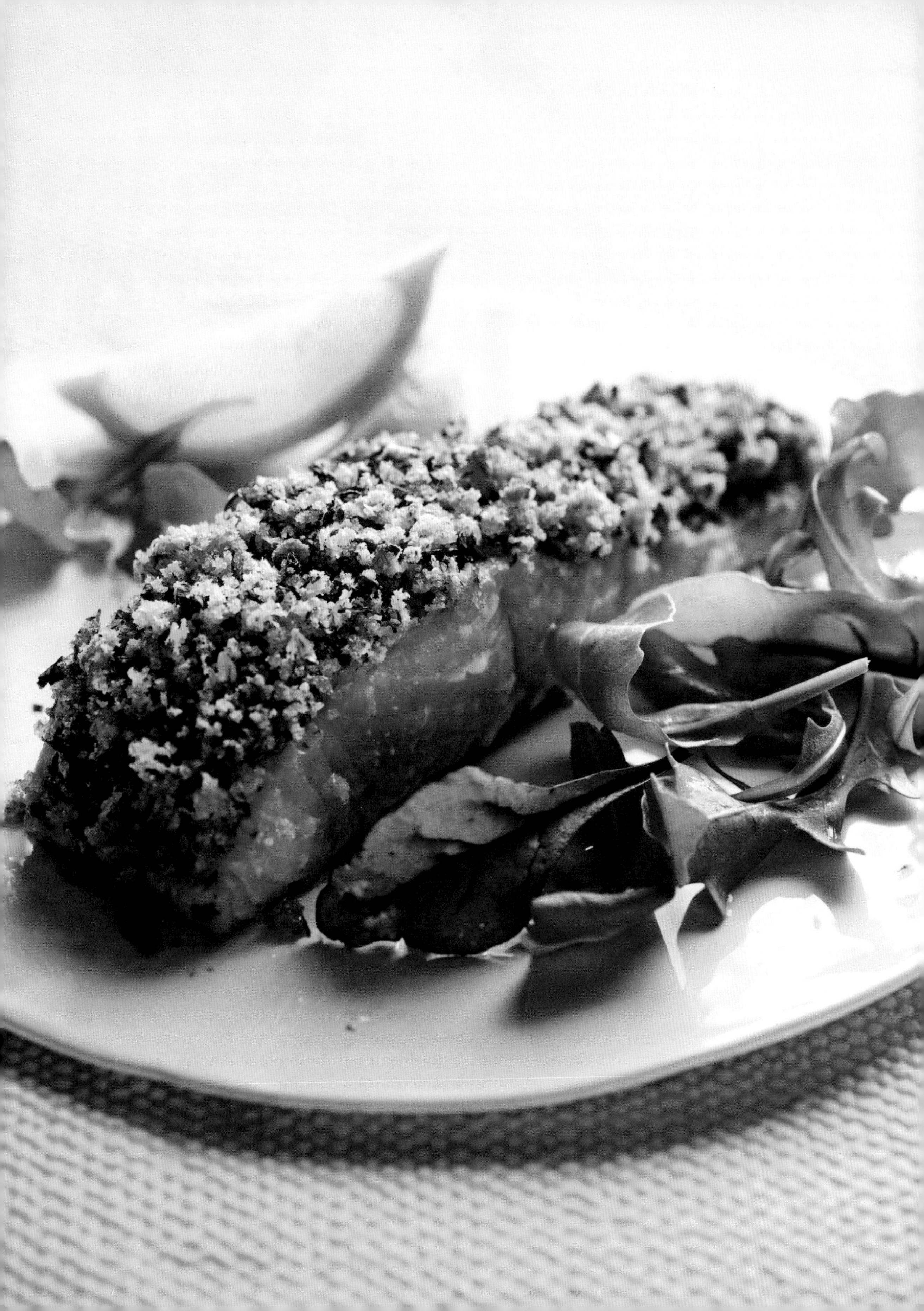

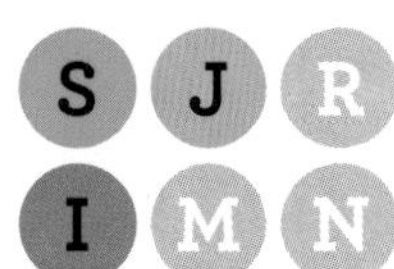

SKIN *Acne*
JOINTS & BONES *Arthritis*
IMMUNE SYSTEM *Colds & flu*
HEART & CIRCULATION
High blood pressure, High cholesterol, Heart disease

Immune-boosting jumbo shrimp curry

I've always loved shrimp—they're fantastic for the health of the skin, and also for the immune system. I'm a curry freak too, so this dish is heaven for me.

SERVES 2 TO 3

1 large onion, coarsely chopped
4 garlic cloves, minced
1 red chili pepper, coarsely chopped
olive oil, for cooking
1-inch piece fresh gingerroot, peeled and coarsely chopped
sea salt
1½ cups cherry tomatoes, coarsely chopped
2 teaspoons mild curry powder
1 teaspoon turmeric
½ teaspoon ground cumin
1 teaspoon ground coriander
1 teaspoon garam masala
1 pound raw peeled jumbo shrimp
3 tablespoons live probiotic plain yogurt
½ teaspoon ground cinnamon
small handful fresh cilantro leaves, coarsely chopped (optional)

Put the onion, garlic, and chopped chili pepper in a small blender or food processor and process to a fine purée.

Heat a little olive oil in a large pan, add the onion purée and the chopped ginger, season with salt, and cook for about 10 minutes, or until the purée has changed color. It will get much darker in color and become less pungent in both taste and aroma.

Once the purée has reached this stage, add the cherry tomatoes and all the spices except the cinnamon. Continue to cook for another 10 minutes, stirring frequently.

Add the jumbo shrimp and the yogurt and cook for another 10 minutes, stirring frequently.

At this stage, stir in the cinnamon and garnish with the chopped cilantro, if using. Serve with cooked quinoa and a green salad, if you like.

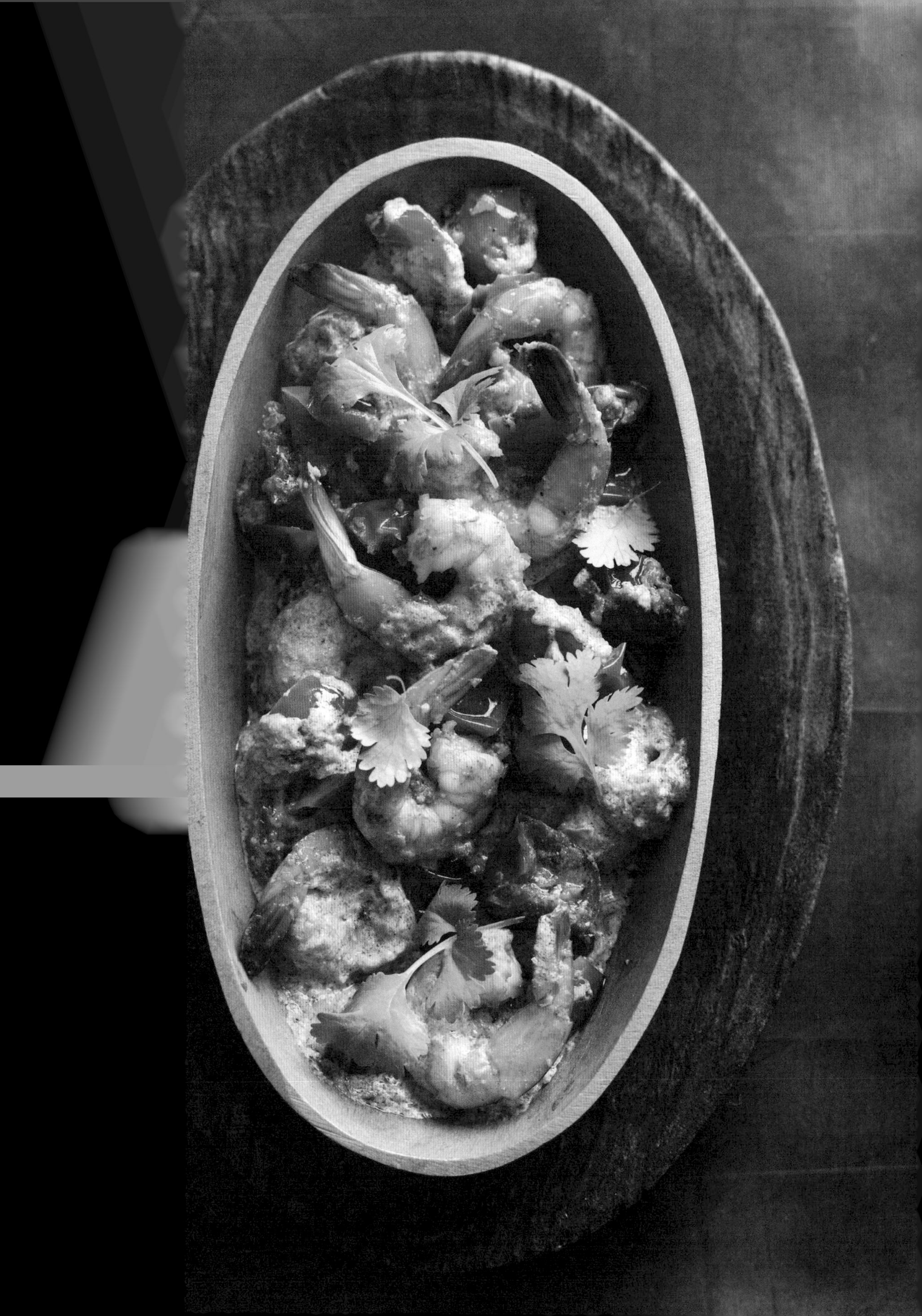

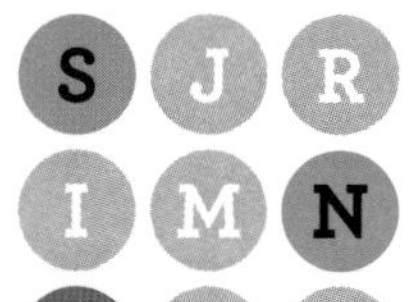

SKIN *Acne*
MENTAL HEALTH & NERVOUS SYSTEM *Insomnia*
HEART & CIRCULATION *High blood pressure, High cholesterol*

Oat-crusted tuna steak with asparagus purée

I sometimes pull this dish out of the bag at dinner parties, as it looks good and has a wonderful, sophisticated flavor—not to mention the fact that it really does you good.

SERVES 2

olive oil, for greasing and cooking
1 small onion, minced
½ bunch asparagus, trimmed
sea salt and black pepper
5 tablespoons rolled oats
2 tablespoons grated Parmesan cheese
2 tuna steaks, about 5 ounces each

Preheat the oven to 400°F and line a baking sheet with aluminum foil, then grease it lightly with oil.

Heat a little olive oil in a pan, add the onion, and cook for 5 to 8 minutes, or until soft and translucent. Add the asparagus and cook for another minute, then add enough water to just cover it. Simmer for about 10 minutes, or until the asparagus has softened and turned bright green. Season with salt and pepper, transfer to a food processor and process to a thick purée.

In a shallow bowl, mix the oats and Parmesan, season with salt and pepper, and mix together thoroughly. Press the tuna steaks lightly into the oat mixture, and turn to make sure they are well covered. Place the steaks on the baking sheet and bake in the oven for 15 to 20 minutes, or until golden brown.

Warm the asparagus purée gently in a small pan. Place each tuna steak in the center of a plate and pour the asparagus purée around it.

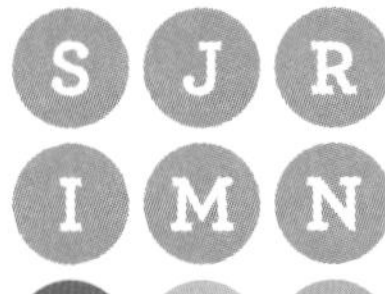

HEART & CIRCULATION *High blood pressure*
DIGESTIVE SYSTEM
REPRODUCTIVE & URINARY SYSTEMS *Problematic periods*

Broiled mackerel fillet with sautéed fennel and leek

This is a gorgeous dinner, bursting with masses of nutrients. It will keep you full, but is still light.

SERVES 2

- 2 fresh mackerel fillets, about 5 ounces each
- olive oil, for cooking
- sea salt and black pepper
- 1 garlic clove, minced
- 1 red chili pepper, minced
- 1 large leek, thinly sliced
- 2 small fennel bulbs, cut into thin strips
- 8 cherry tomatoes
- 1 lemon, cut into wedges, to serve

Preheat the broiler. Place the mackerel fillet on a baking sheet, season with salt and pepper, broil for 5 to 7 minutes, until golden and thoroughly cooked.

Heat a little olive oil in a pan, add the garlic and chili pepper, and cook over low heat for about 1 minute. Add the leek and fennel, and cook for 2 minutes. Add the cherry tomatoes and continue to cook until the leek and fennel are soft and the tomatoes are just starting to split, 3 to 6 minutes. Season with salt and pepper.

Pile some sautéed leek and fennel in the center of each plate. Place the broiled mackerel on top and add a lemon wedge. Serve immediately, with some boiled new potatoes if you like.

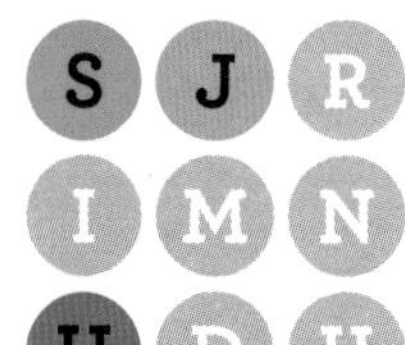

SKIN *Acne, Eczema, Psoriasis*
JOINTS & BONES *Arthritis, Bursitis*
HEART & CIRCULATION *High cholesterol*

Broiled salmon with spinach and spiced carrot mash

I got the inspiration for this from a dish I often eat at my favorite hotel in Dublin, Ireland, whenever work takes me there. Their slightly more rib-sticking version made me fall in love with spiced carrot mash. A match made in heaven.

SERVES 2

5 large carrots, sliced
sea salt and black pepper
2 large salmon fillets, about 5 ounces each
2 large handfuls spinach
small piece of butter
½ teaspoon mixed spice
2 sprigs fresh parsley leaves, minced
lemon wedges, to serve

Put the carrots in a small pan and cover with water. Bring to a boil, then reduce the heat and simmer for 10 to 15 minutes, or until tender. An even better option, if possible, is to steam them, which retains more nutrients.

Preheat the broiler. Season the salmon fillets and put them on a baking sheet and broil for 8 to 10 minutes, or until they begin to turn golden brown, turning them once during cooking.

Put the spinach in a pan with a few tablespoons water, place over high heat, and cook, covered, for 3 to 4 minutes, or until wilted. Drain well.

Drain the cooked carrots and place them in a large bowl. Mash them with a potato masher. Add the butter and mixed spice, season with salt and pepper, and mash again until smooth. Stir in the chopped parsley. To assemble, put the spinach in the center of a plate, place the broiled salmon on top, and add the mash next to it. Serve with lemon wedges.

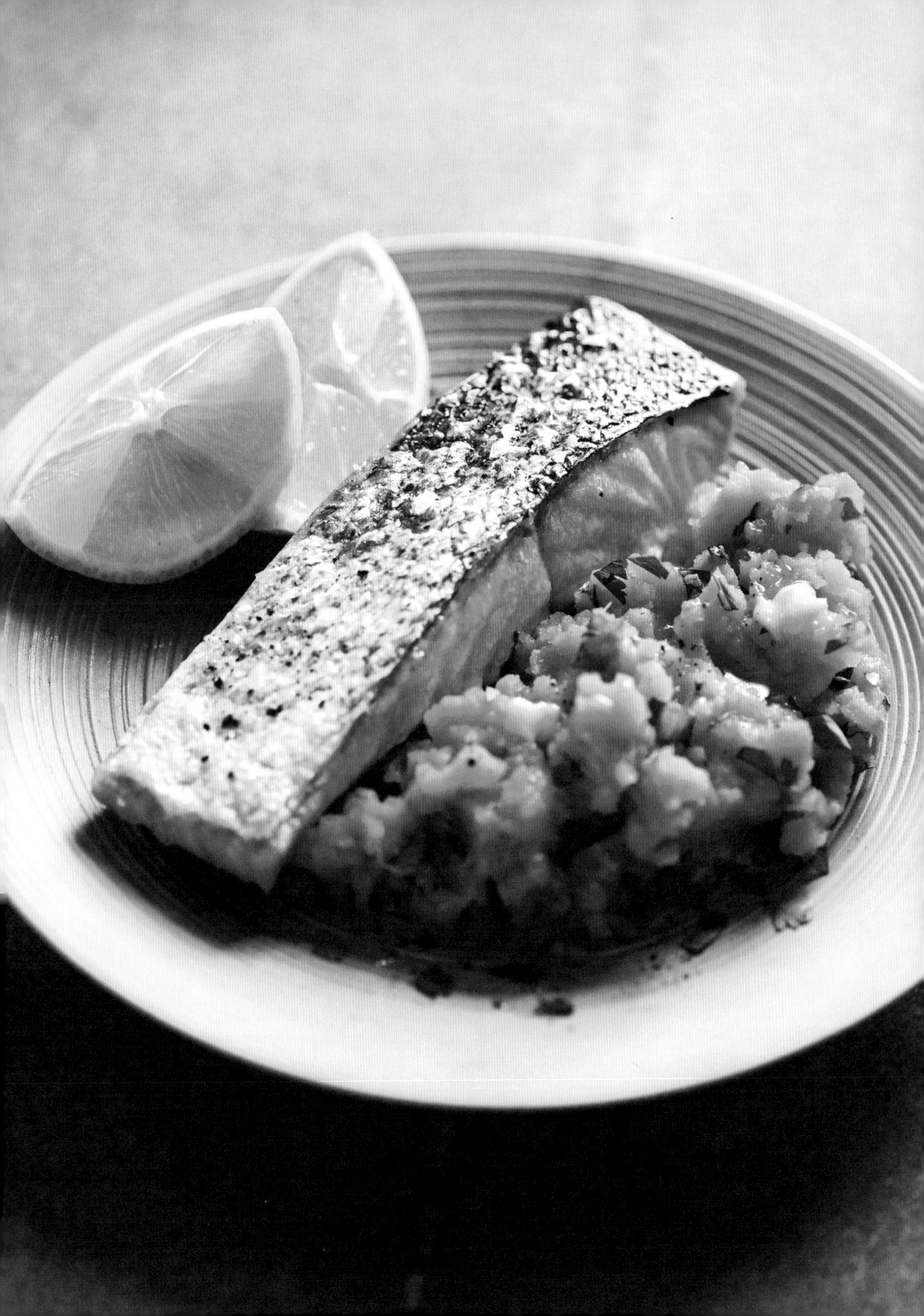

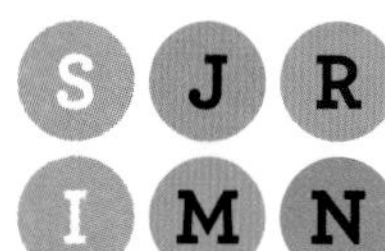

JOINTS & BONES *Arthritis*
RESPIRATORY SYSTEM *Asthma*
METABOLIC SYSTEM *Diabetes (Type 2)*
MENTAL HEALTH & NERVOUS SYSTEM *Anxiety, Depression*
HEART & CIRCULATION *High blood pressure, High cholesterol*

Mackerel marinated with beet and horseradish

I know this sounds like a weird combination, but trust me, it's a marriage made in heaven. Red beets and horseradish is a classic combination, and the intense flavor of the mackerel takes the whole thing to another level. Try it—you'll be glad you did!

SERVES 2

- 2 large cooked red beets
- 4 teaspoons prepared horseradish
- 1 tablespoon live probiotic plain yogurt
- juice of ½ lemon
- 2 mackerel fillets, about 5 ounces each
- sea salt and black pepper

Make the marinade by placing the beets, horseradish, yogurt, and lemon juice in a food processor, then process to a smooth purée.

Put the marinade in a bowl or dish, add the mackerel fillets, and make sure that they are well covered in the marinade. Let marinate in the refrigerator for 2 to 3 hours.

Once marinated, preheat the oven to 375°F and line a baking sheet with aluminum foil. Put the mackerel on the prepared sheet and bake in the oven for about 8 minutes, or until just cooked through. To check, insert the tip of a knife into the center of a fillet: the flesh should flake and no longer look translucent.

Serve with roasted vegetables, quinoa, salad, or even in a wrap.

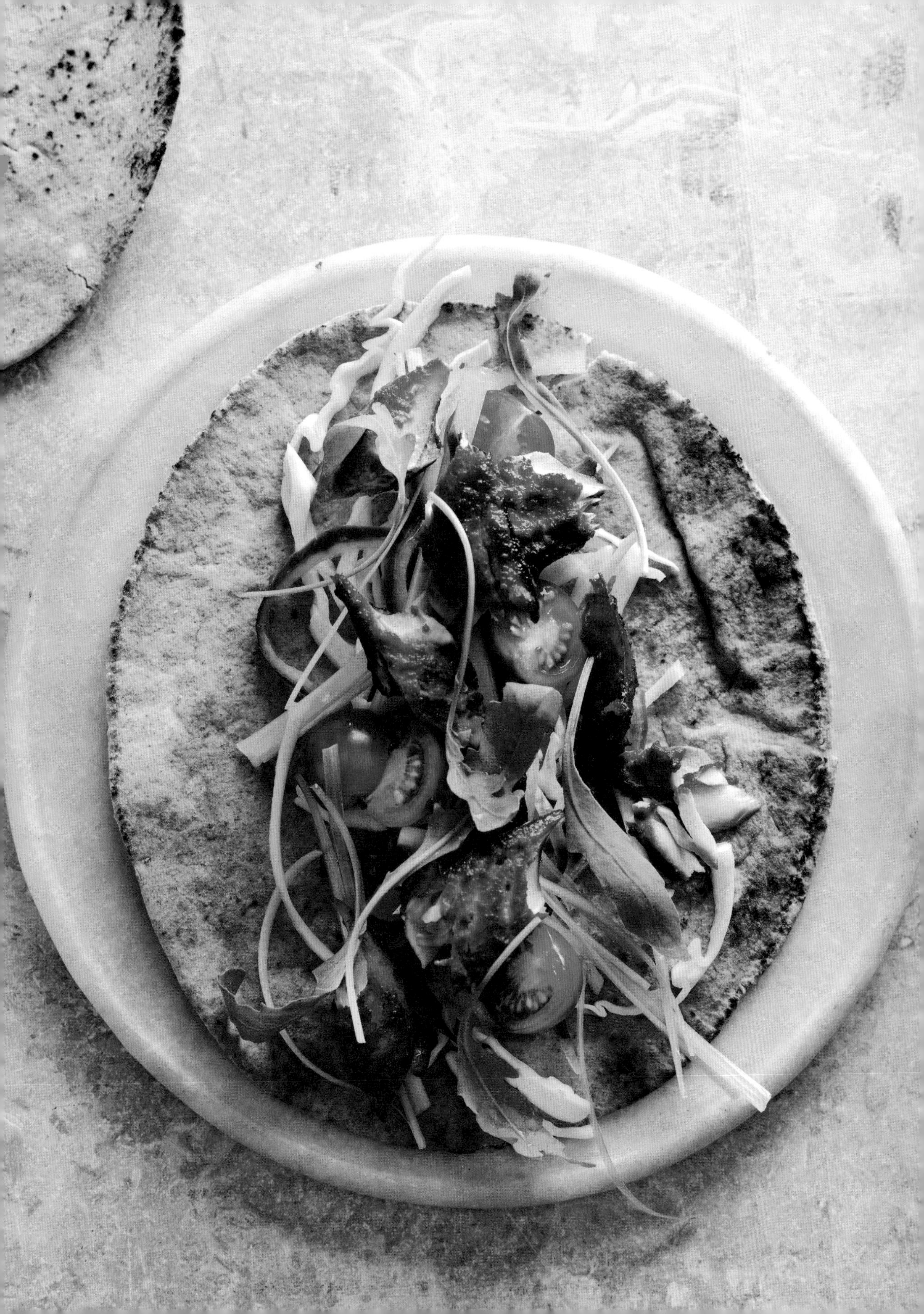

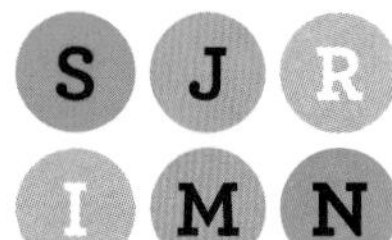

SKIN *Acne, Eczema*
JOINTS & BONES *Arthritis*
METABOLIC SYSTEM *Diabetes (Type 2)*
MENTAL HEALTH & NERVOUS SYSTEM *Anxiety, Depression, Stress*
REPRODUCTIVE & URINARY SYSTEMS *Polycystic ovary syndrome*

Salmon and jumbo shrimp skewers with citrus quinoa salad

This dish is gorgeous and feels very summery. It delivers masses of minerals, fatty acids, and protein, too, as well as all sorts of other goodies. That's got to be good! Ask at the fish counter to have the fish skinned.

SERVES 1 TO 2

- 1 salmon fillet (about 5 ounces), skinned and cut into cubes
- 4 ounces raw peeled jumbo shrimp
- sea salt and black pepper
- generous ½ cup quinoa
- 2 teaspoons vegetable stock powder, or 1 vegetable stock cube
- handful fresh parsley leaves, minced
- grated zest and juice of 1 lime

Bring a pan of water to a boil and add the quinoa. Add a couple teaspoons of vegetable stock powder or a vegetable stock cube to the water to give greater depth of flavor, and cook for 10 to 15 minutes. When cooked, the grains should look translucent and have little white tails on the side.

Preheat the broiler. Take some pre-soaked wooden or metal skewers and thread alternating cubes of salmon and jumbo shrimp onto them. Season with salt and pepper. Place under the broiler for about 10 minutes, turning them 2 to 3 times.

Place the cooked quinoa into a bowl and stir in the chopped parsley. Add the zest and juice of the lime. Season with salt and pepper and stir well.

Put some of the quinoa salad onto serving plates and place the cooked skewers on top. Serve with an arugula salad.

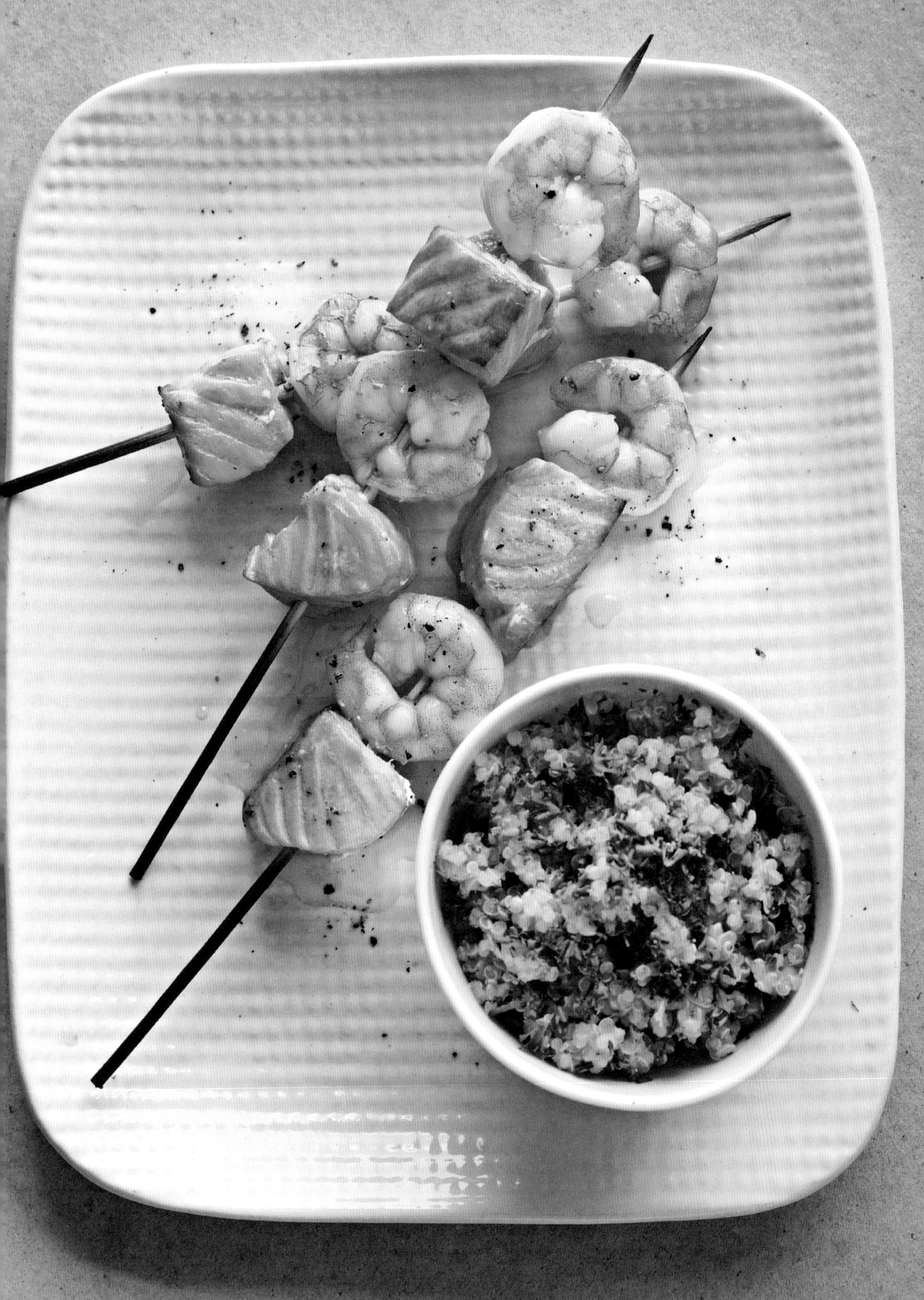

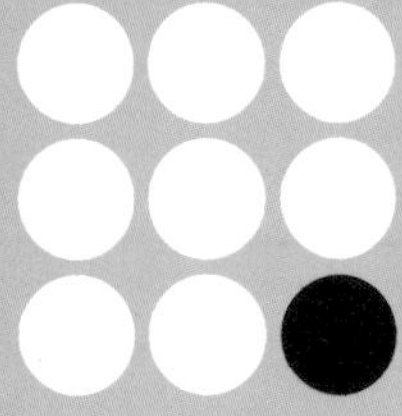

Sweet treats

Many people think a healthy diet has to involve self-flagellation and suffering, and that sweet treats and goodies are completely off the menu. Well, forget that, I say! A life without enjoyment is a pretty miserable one, and if you adopt that attitude you'll soon end up falling off the wagon and going back to your old ways of eating. With a bit of imagination and a smart choice of ingredients, it is possible to have your cake and eat it: you really can make sweet treats that actually benefit your health.

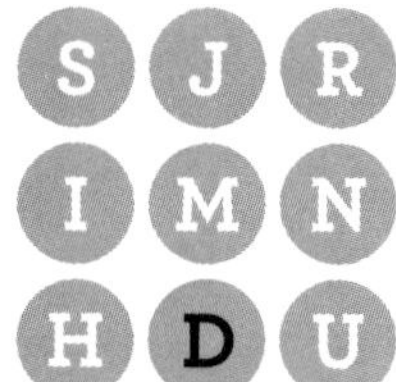

Probiotic pineapple, papaya, and mint frozen yogurt Homemade frozen yogurts and sorbets are actually pretty easy, if you have some time on your hands. This one is lovely and fresh.

SERVES 2 TO 3

1 small, ripe pineapple
1 small, ripe papaya
handful fresh mint leaves
1 tablespoon honey
generous 2 cups live probiotic plain yogurt

Peel the pineapple by slicing off each end, then slicing downward between the skin and the flesh with a sharp knife. Remove and discard the skin, and remove the spiky brown dots, or "eyes," from the flesh with the tip of the knife. Cut the flesh into rough chunks and place them in a food processor. Halve the papaya, scoop out the seeds, then scoop the flesh into the processor.

Chop the mint leaves and add them, along with the honey and yogurt. Process on high speed to create a creamy mixture that resembles a smoothie. Transfer this mixture to a tub, or freezerproof pan or dish, and place in the freezer. After 30 minutes, the edges of the mixture should have started to freeze. Mix thoroughly with a fork to break up the frozen pieces, and return to the freezer for another 30 minutes. Alternatively, process briefly in a food processor and return to the freezer.

After 30 minutes, remove and repeat the process. Continue doing this for 2 to 3 hours, or until an ice-cream texture is reached.

If you like, you can churn the mixture in an ice-cream machine, following the manufacturer's instructions, then transfer to the freezer.

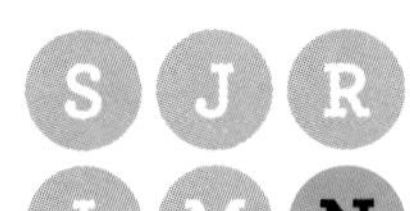
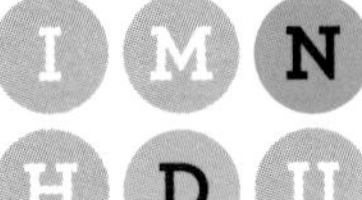

MENTAL HEALTH & NERVOUS SYSTEM *Insomnia*
DIGESTIVE SYSTEM *Constipation, Hemorrhoids*

Goodnight spiced cherry crumble

This gorgeous dessert packs quite a nutritional punch, and tastes as though it's far less healthy than it actually is. We all need a little treat!

SERVES 4

- generous 1½ pounds fresh or frozen cherries, thawed if frozen
- 1 tablespoon honey
- generous 1 cup rolled oats
- ¾ cup whole wheat flour
- 1 teaspoon ground cinnamon
- 1 tablespoon good quality cane sugar
- 1 tablespoon light olive oil
- live probiotic plain yogurt, to serve

Preheat the oven to 350°F. Remove the stems and pits from the cherries. You can split them in half and just pull the pits out.

Place the pitted cherries in a small pan with about 1 tablespoon water and the honey. Simmer over high heat for 4 to 5 minutes, or until the cherries begin to soften and turn into a jammy mush.

Combine the oats, flour, cinnamon, and sugar with the olive oil in a bowl. Mix well to create a bread crumb-like texture.

Place the cherry mixture in a small baking dish. Top with the crumble mixture and bake in the oven for about 30 minutes, or until golden brown. Let cool for a few minutes before serving with yogurt.

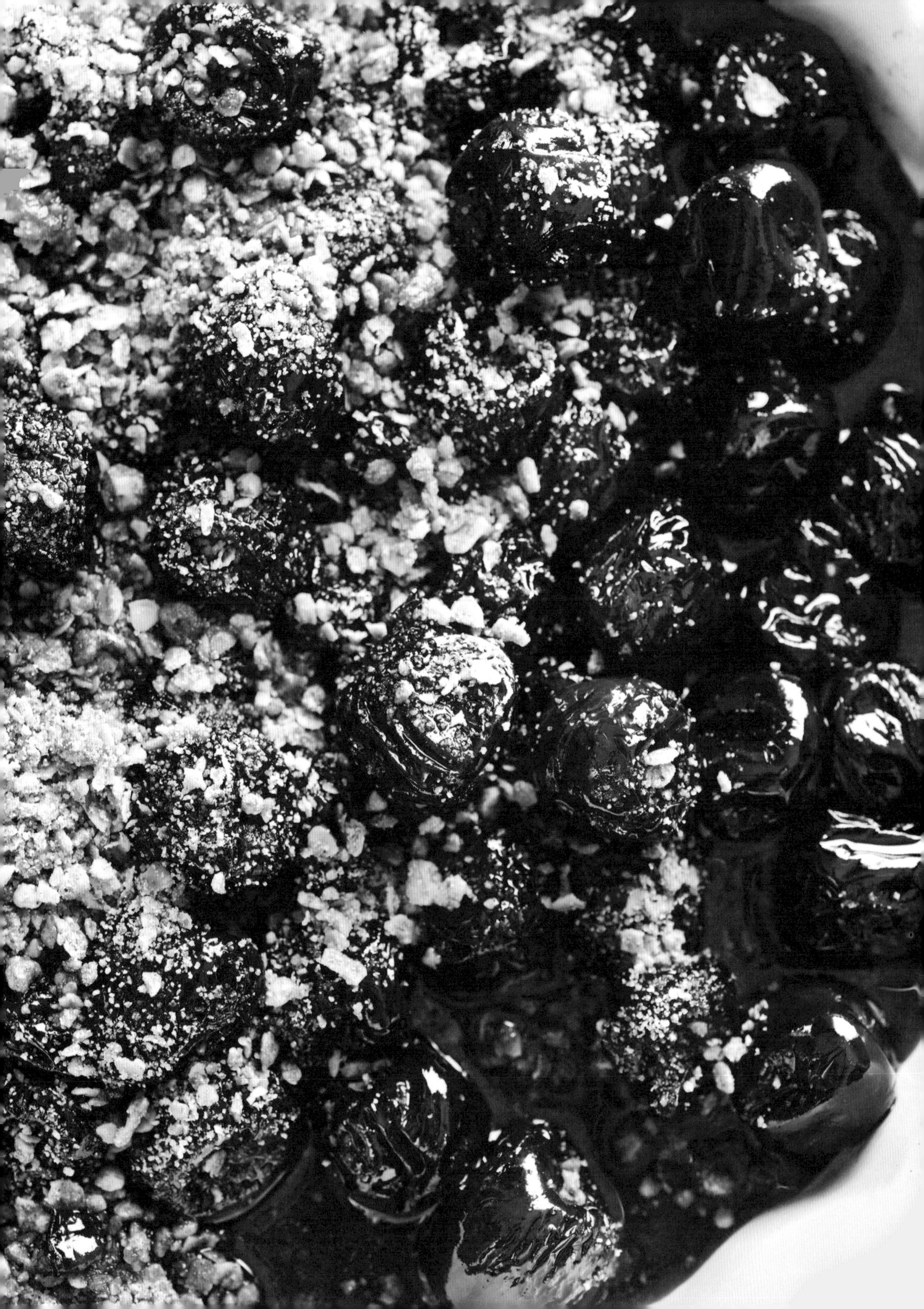

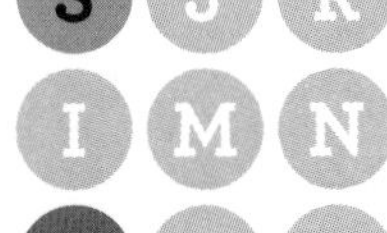

SKIN *Eczema*
HEART & CIRCULATION *High cholesterol, High blood pressure*

Mint chocolate no-cheese cake

This lovely dessert takes a little bit of effort, but the results are amazing—the cheesecake-torte effect will shock your friends, especially if you wait until afterward to tell them what's in it!

SERVES 6 TO 8

For the base:
1⅓ cups mixed nuts (such as walnuts, brazil nuts, and hazelnuts)
6 pitted dates
3 tablespoons coconut oil

For the chocolate layer:
4 very ripe, very soft avocados
5 tablespoons good quality unsweetened cocoa (preferably raw cacao powder)
4 tablespoons honey, or to taste
½-1 teaspoon peppermint extract
3 tablespoons coconut oil, melted
fresh mint leaves, to decorate (optional)

To make the base, put the nuts and dates in a food processor and process at full speed until a stiff dough has formed. Melt the coconut oil gently in a small pan over low heat and add the melted oil to the mixture. Process again until well mixed. Transfer the mixture to a 9-inch spring form pan, and line the bottom with it, pressing down firmly with the back of the spoon to create a tightly compressed layer in the pan. Put the pan in the freezer to set while you begin preparing the chocolate layer.

Halve the avocados, remove the pits, and scoop the flesh into the cleaned food processor. Add the unsweetened cocoa, honey, peppermint extract, and melted coconut oil, and blend to make a thick, velvety chocolate mousse.

Remove from the freezer and pour the chocolate mixture over the base, then smooth down into an even layer with a palette knife. Chill in the refrigerator for at least 5 hours before serving. This will allow the coconut oil to set to create a firm base, and a velvety, torte-like topping. Decorate with mint leaves before serving, if you like.

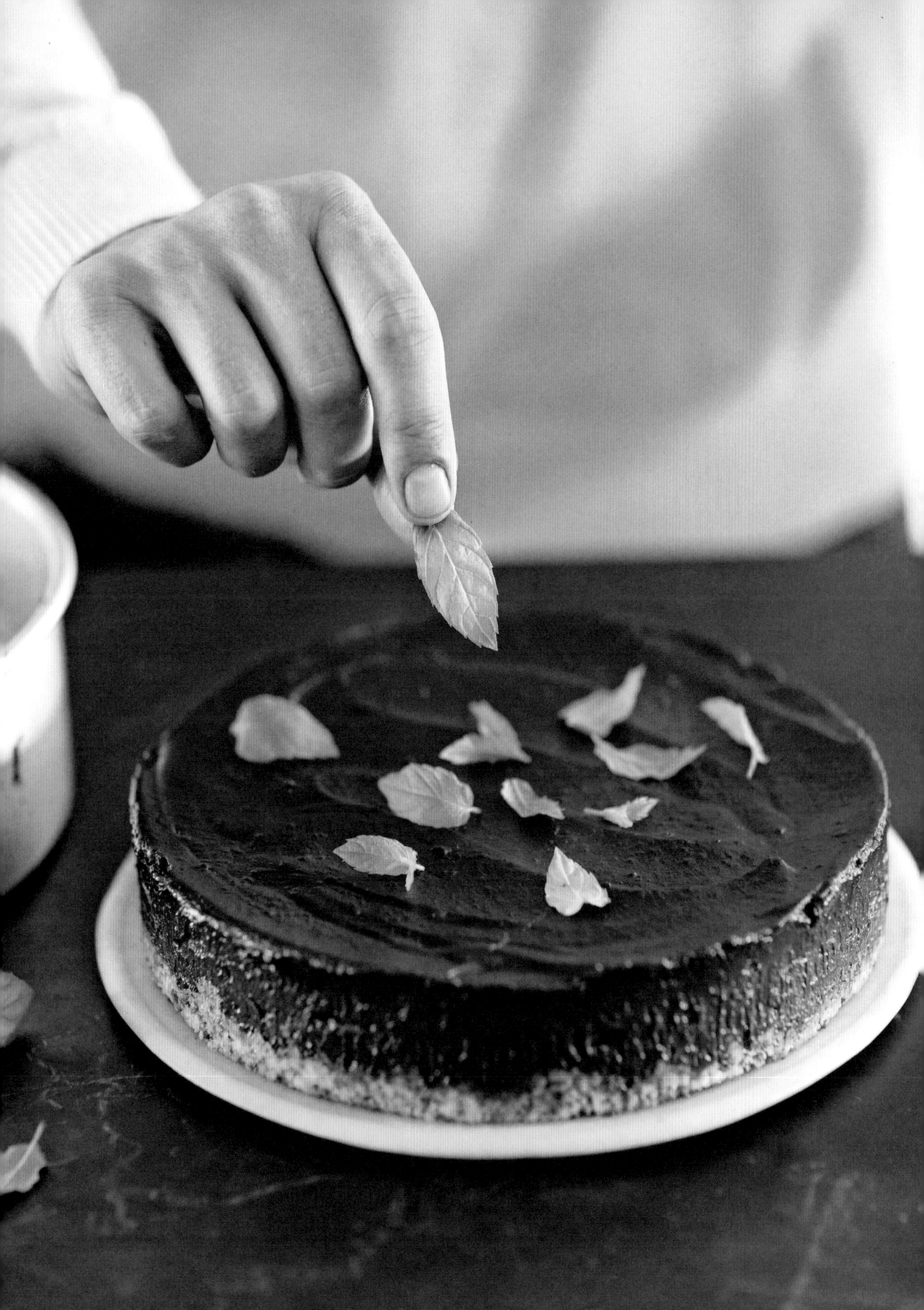

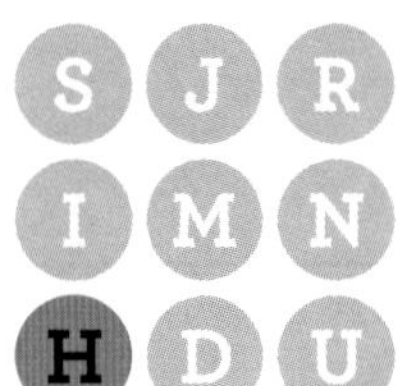

Baked spiced apple wedges with heart-healthy compote

This is a lovely, summery dessert that's sweetly satisfying, yet incredibly virtuous.

SERVES 2 TO 3

2 Golden Delicious apples
2 teaspoons maple syrup
1 teaspoon ground cinnamon
1 cup fresh blueberries
½ red chili pepper, seeded and minced
handful pecan nuts, roughly chopped, to serve (optional)
live probiotic plain yogurt, to serve

Preheat the oven to 400°F. Cut the apples into eighths, without peeling them, and remove the seeds and fibrous part around the seeds.

Place the apple wedges on a baking sheet and bake in the oven for 15 minutes. Remove the tray from the oven, drizzle the wedges with maple syrup, and sprinkle with cinnamon. Return to the oven for another 15 to 20 minutes, or until soft and bubbling.

To make the blueberry compote, place the blueberries in a pan with 1 tablespoon water and the chili pepper. Cook over high heat for 4 to 5 minutes, or until the blueberries begin to release their juices and break down into a compote. Pour the compote over the baked apple wedges and sprinkle with the chopped pecans, if using. Serve with a dollop of yogurt.

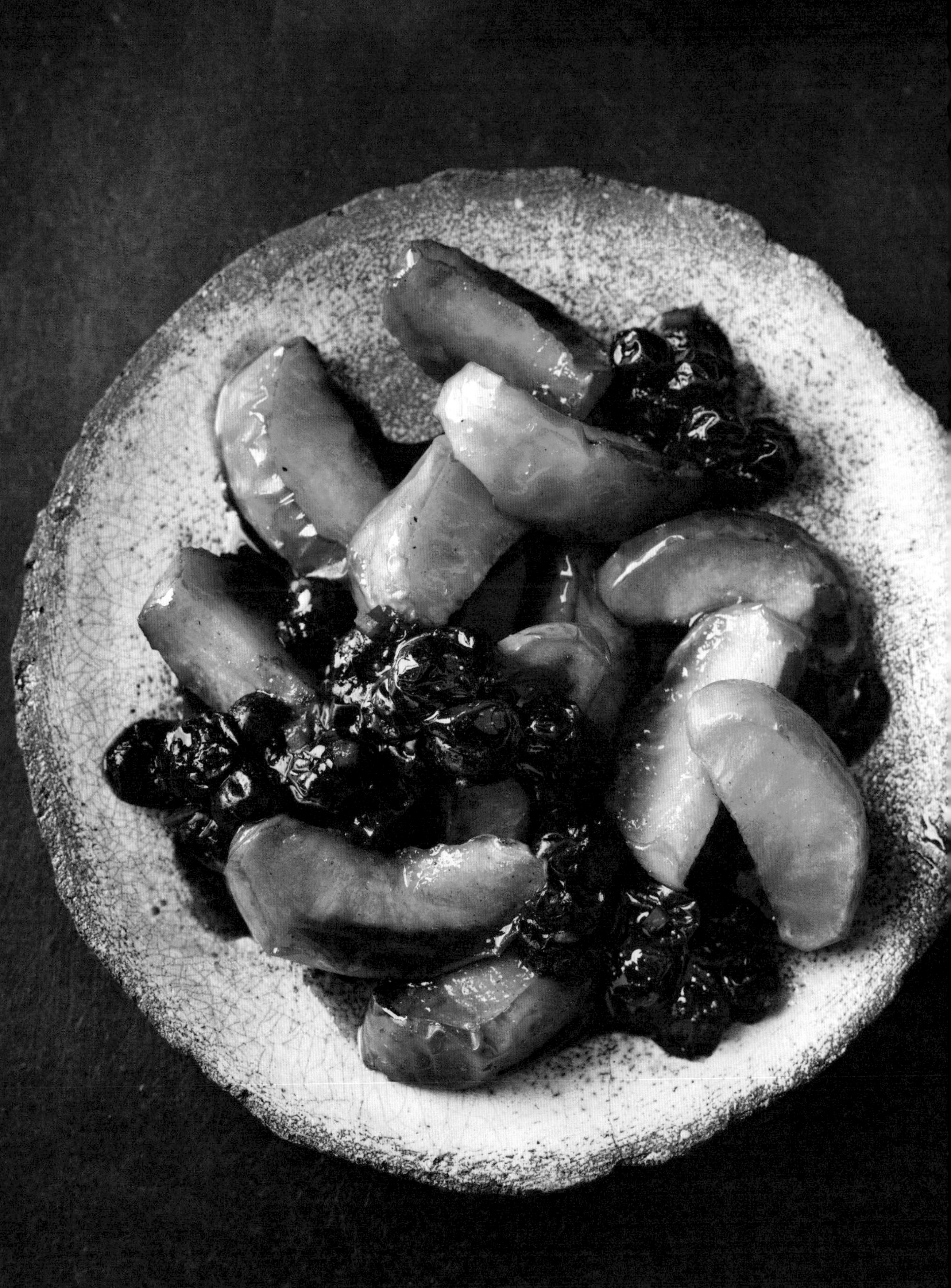

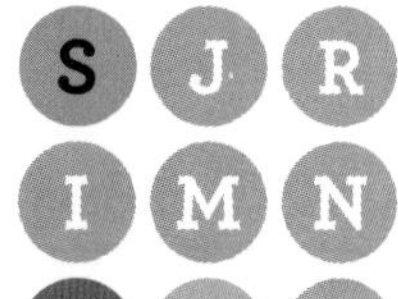

SKIN *Eczema*
HEART & CIRCULATION *High blood pressure, High cholesterol*
DIGESTIVE SYSTEM *Cramp*

Cheating chocolate-orange delight

This dish is an awesome example of how you really can have your cake and eat it. It has fooled even the most hardcore of chocaholics, and, hands down, they just don't believe me when I tell them the ingredients. Use raw cacao powder if you can find it—it's available in many health food stores.

SERVES 2 TO 3

2 very ripe avocados
finely grated zest and juice of 1 large orange
1 tablespoon honey
3 tablespoons good quality cocoa or cacao powder

Halve the avocados, discarding the pits. Scoop out the flesh with a spoon and put it in a food processor. Add the remaining ingredients and process to make a thick, rich, mousse-like dessert.

You can add extra cocoa powder or honey to make it sweeter or more chocolatey, if you like. Serve in a cocktail glass or ramekin.

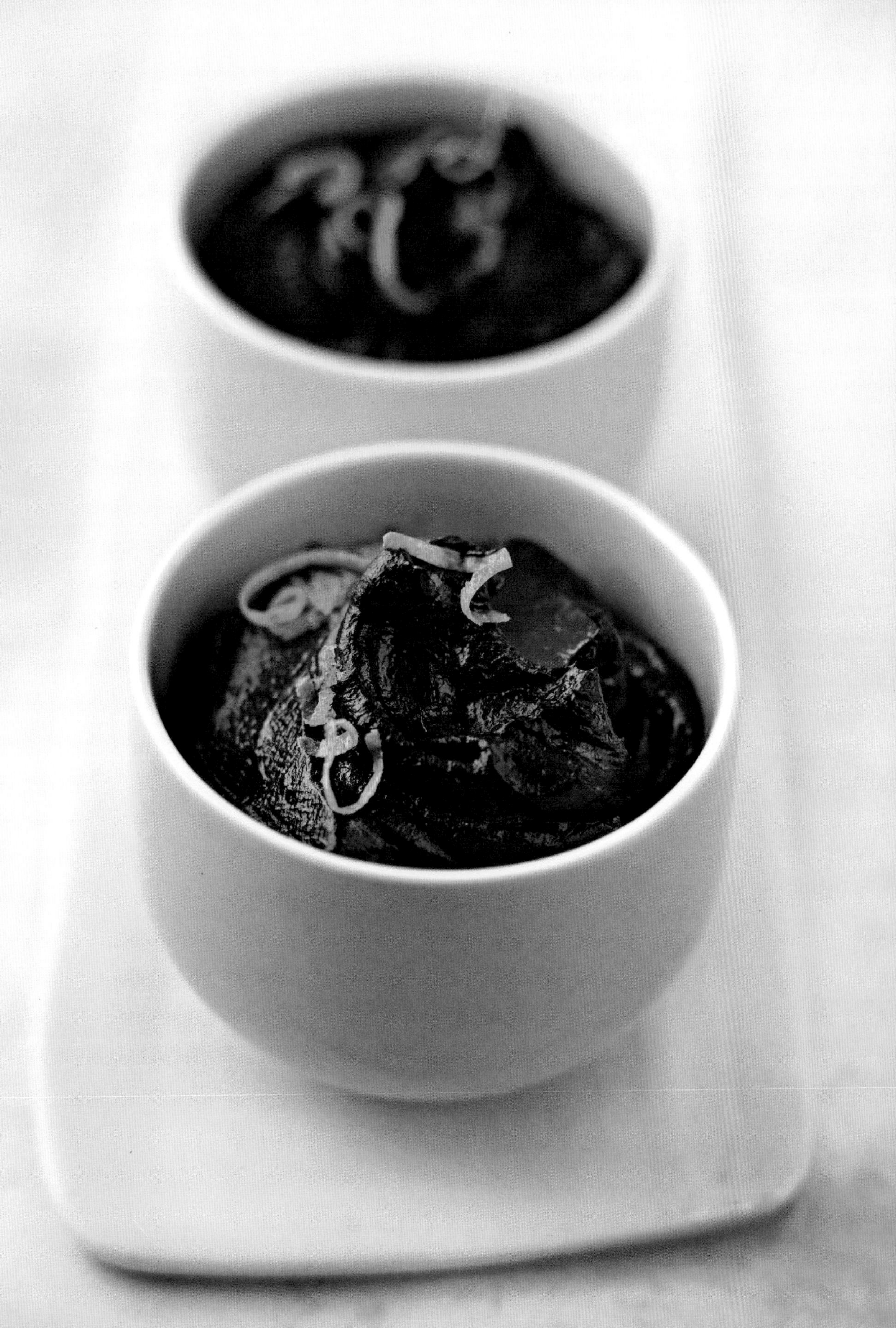

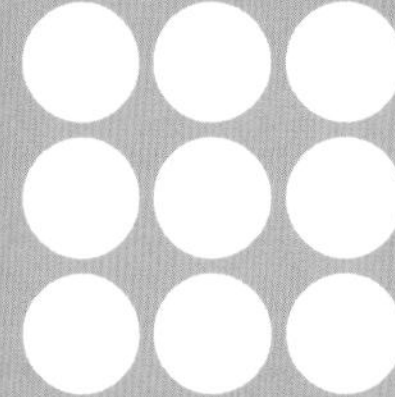

Drinks

It's not all about what we eat; what we drink matters too. It's very easy to reach for unhealthy options like sugary sodas. The best drink of all for us is water, but it's easy to make some powerful health-giving drinks that can add to your health regime. Here are a few of my favorites. A couple of them require a juicer—these gadgets were once pricey and tricky to use, but they're now reasonably priced and easy to use and clean.

Chocolate for breakfast: hurrah! Chocolate is often given a bad rap, but this isn't always justified. Take away the sugar, cream, and all the other gunk that is added to chocolate bars, and you are actually left with a very nutritious ingredient indeed. And the banana berry smoothie is another quick, easy smoothie that makes a great nutrient-packed breakfast.

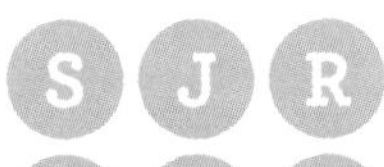

DIGESTIVE SYSTEM

Banana berry smoothie

SERVES 1 TO 2

2 ripe bananas
1 cup frozen mixed berries
2/3 cup live probiotic plain yogurt
scant 1/2 cup orange or apple juice

Place all the ingredients in a blender and process to make a thick, creamy smoothie.

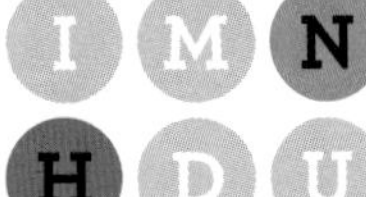

JOINTS & BONES *Osteoporosis*
MENTAL HEALTH & NERVOUS SYSTEM *Anxiety*
HEART & CIRCULATION *High blood pressure*

Chocolate morning smoothie

SERVES 1

generous 1 cup milk, or soy or almond milk
1 banana
2 tablespoons good quality pure unsweetened cocoa (preferably raw cacao powder)
2 teaspoons honey

Put all the ingredients in a blender and process to make a thick, luscious, and chocolaty smoothie. Enjoy!

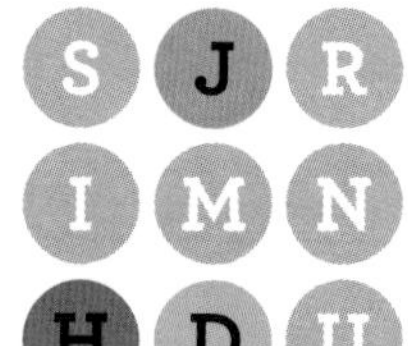

JOINTS & BONES *Arthritis*
HEART & CIRCULATION *High blood pressure*
DIGESTIVE SYSTEM *Bloating, IBS*

Pineapple zing smoothie Guaranteed to put some zing in your thing! OK, I know it may sound like a weird combination of ingredients, but trust me, it really works. The flavors complement each other, and their nutritional benefits do, too. Try it—you'll love it!

SERVES 2 TO 3

½ large ripe pineapple
2 celery stalks, plus the leaves to garnish (optional)
1-inch piece fresh ginger

Peel the pineapple by slicing off each end, then slicing downward between the skin and the flesh with a sharp knife. Remove and discard the skin. Remove the spiky brown dots, or "eyes," from the pineapple flesh with the tip of a small knife, then cut the flesh into chunks and put it in a blender.

Cut the celery into chunks and add it to the blender. Peel the ginger—scraping off the skin with a teaspoon is a good way to do this—and finely chop it, then add to the blender.

Process thoroughly to make a thick, zingy smoothie. You can add a small amount of water to help the ingredients blend, or to make a thinner smoothie, if you prefer.

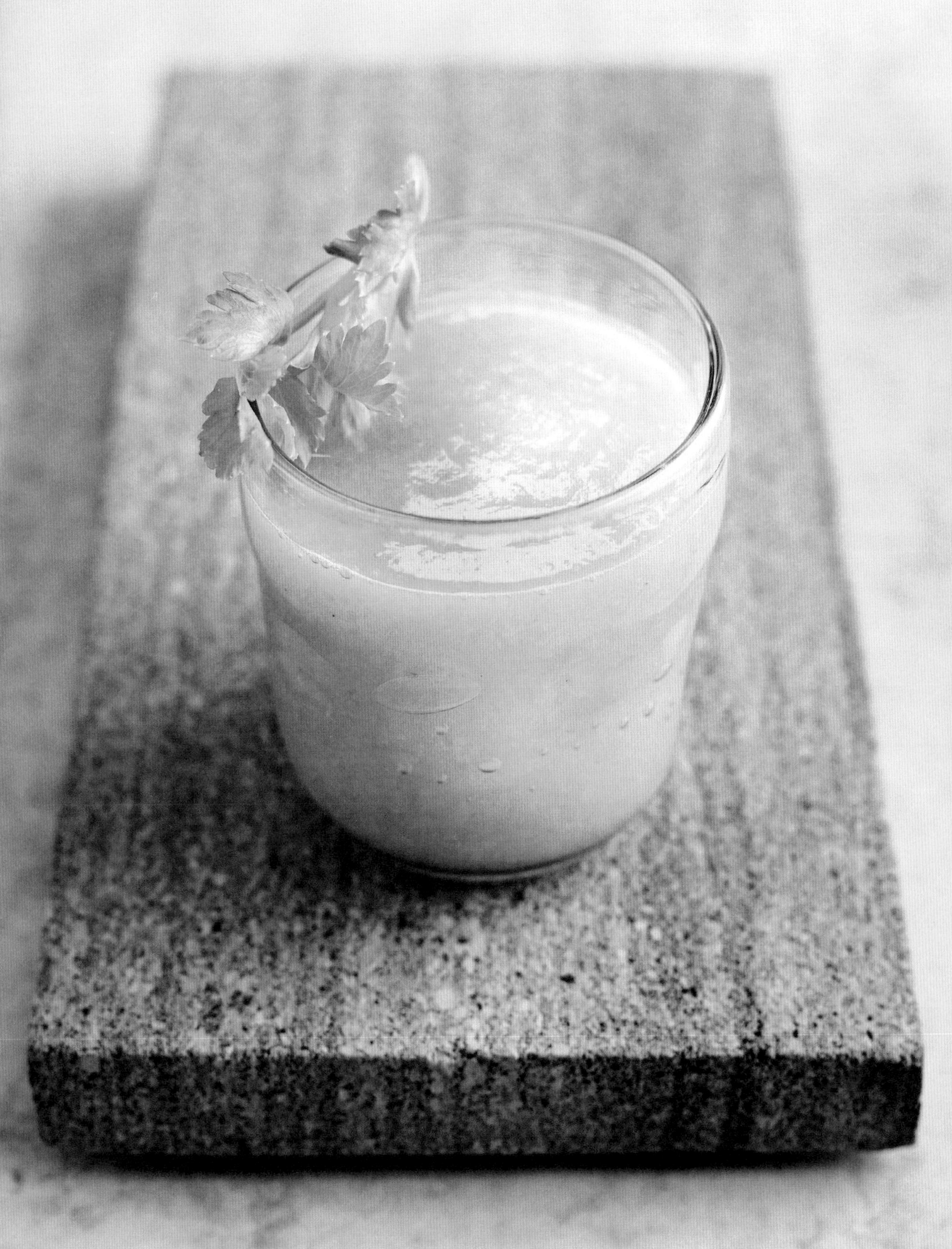

These drinks pack a serious punch, and provide a perfect way to kick-start your day. I'm a big fan of mango lassi and the smoothie is my tribute. The fennel tea used in this recipe is the type you can find in tea bags at any grocery store.

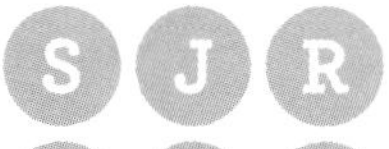

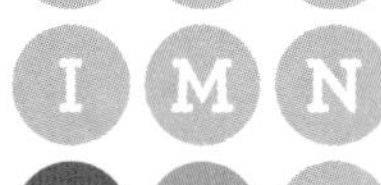

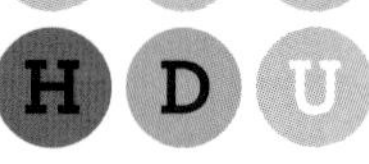

HEART & CIRCULATION
High blood pressure
DIGESTIVE SYSTEM

Wake-up juice

SERVES 1

1 large raw red beet
2 Golden Delicious apples
½-inch piece fresh ginger

Process all the ingredients in a juicer and drink immediately.

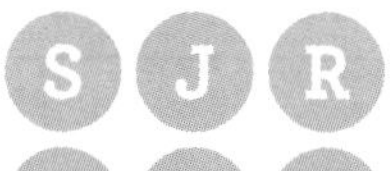

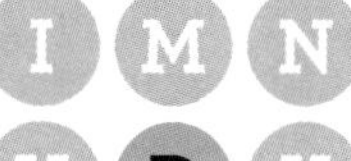

H D U

DIGESTIVE SYSTEM
Bloating, Constipation, IBS

Probiotic mango smoothie

SERVES 1

1 fennel tea bag
1 large, ripe mango, peeled, pitted, and chopped
½ cup live probiotic plain yogurt
1 teaspoon honey

Brew a cup of fennel tea. Leave the bag in the tea and let it cool completely. Measure out ½ cup of the cooled tea and place in a blender.

Place the mango, yogurt, and honey in the blender and process into a smooth, luscious drink.

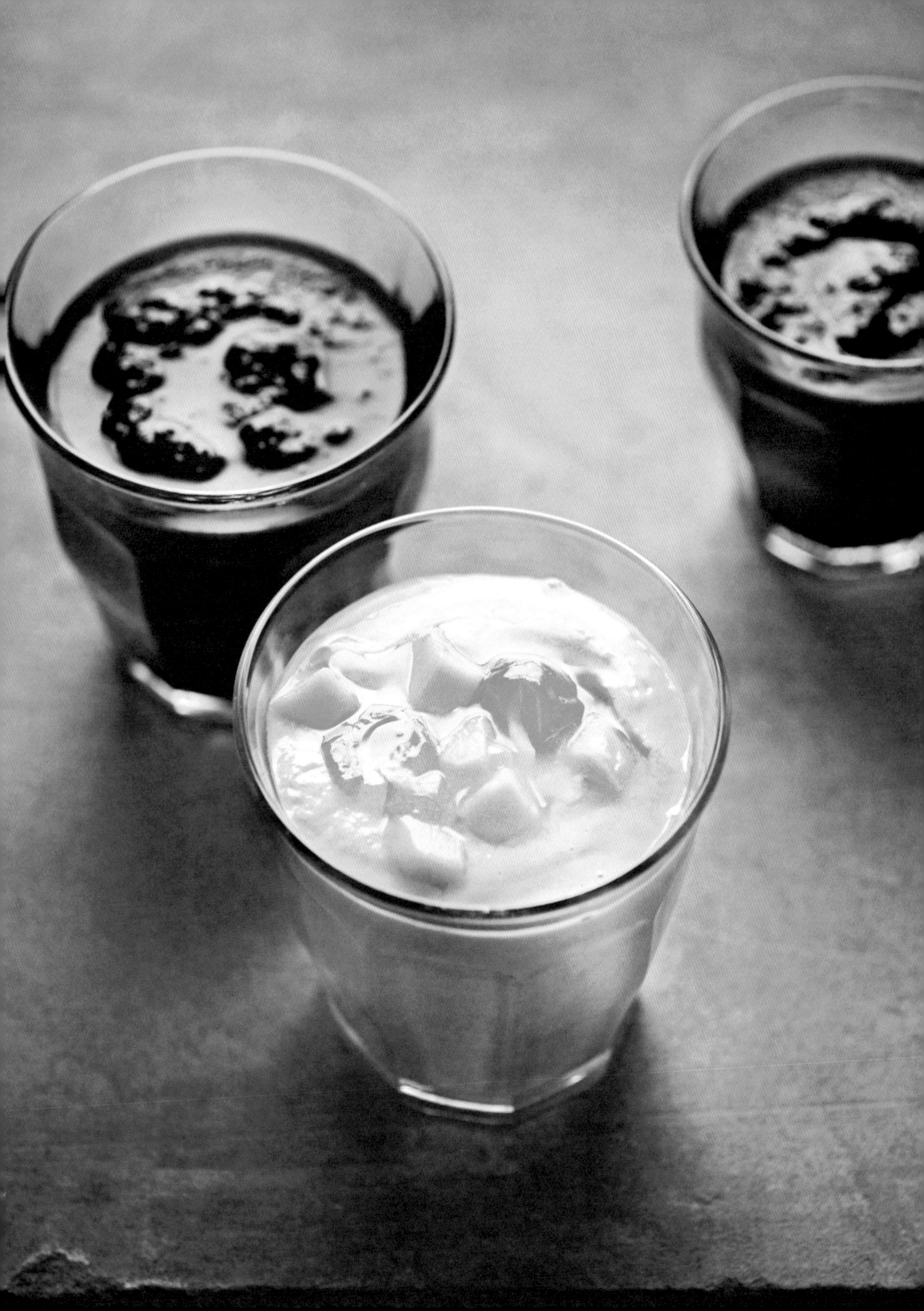

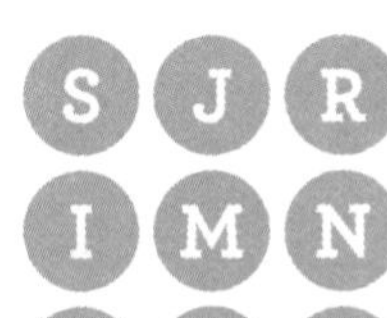

Tummy tea This simple tea tastes wonderful and packs a powerful punch, making it ideal for any digestive issues.

SERVES 1

1 heaping teaspoon fennel seeds
1 heaping teaspoon caraway seeds
1 heaping teaspoon dried mint
handful fresh mint leaves (optional)

Mix the seeds and herbs together and infuse in a mug full of boiling water. Let steep for 10 minutes, then strain and sip.

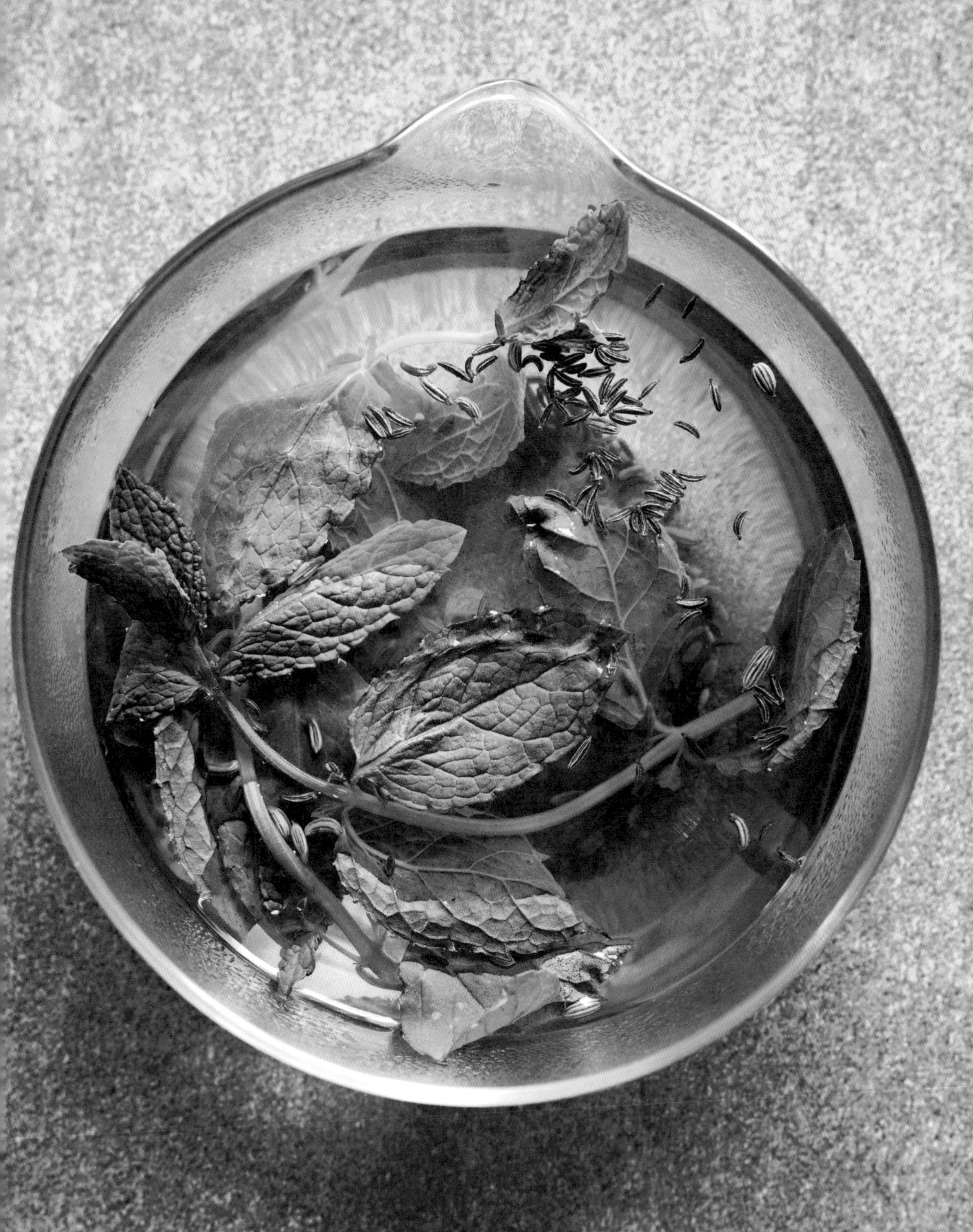

This lovely, simple smoothie takes minutes to make and is a great digestive dynamo and energy tonic! Coconut oil is an easy ingredient to find these days in grocery stores and health food stores. The unusual but delicious pairing of cranberry and celery makes a pungent and powerful juice that's wonderful for the health of the urinary tract.

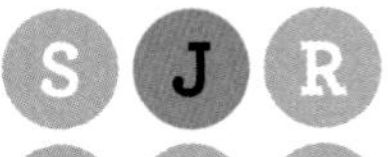

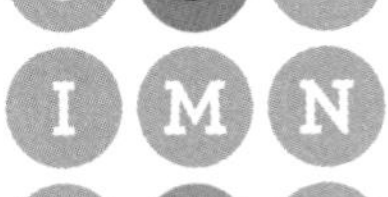

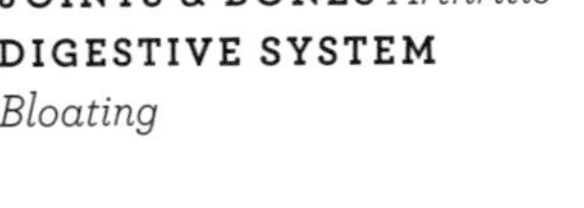

JOINTS & BONES *Arthritis*
DIGESTIVE SYSTEM
Bloating

Sunshine smoothie

SERVES 1 TO 2

1 small, very ripe pineapple, peeled and chopped
1 14-ounce can coconut milk
1 tablespoon coconut oil

Place all the ingredients in a blender, and process into a smooth, luscious drink. Serve over ice.

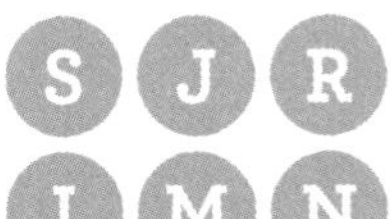

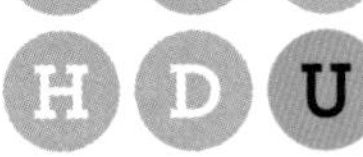

REPRODUCTIVE & URINARY SYSTEMS
Cystitis and other urinary tract infections

Cranberry and celery blast

SERVES 1

1½ cups fresh cranberries
½ Golden Delicious apple, cut into wedges
3 celery stalks

Process all the ingredients in a juicer. Drink immediately.

CONDITIONS

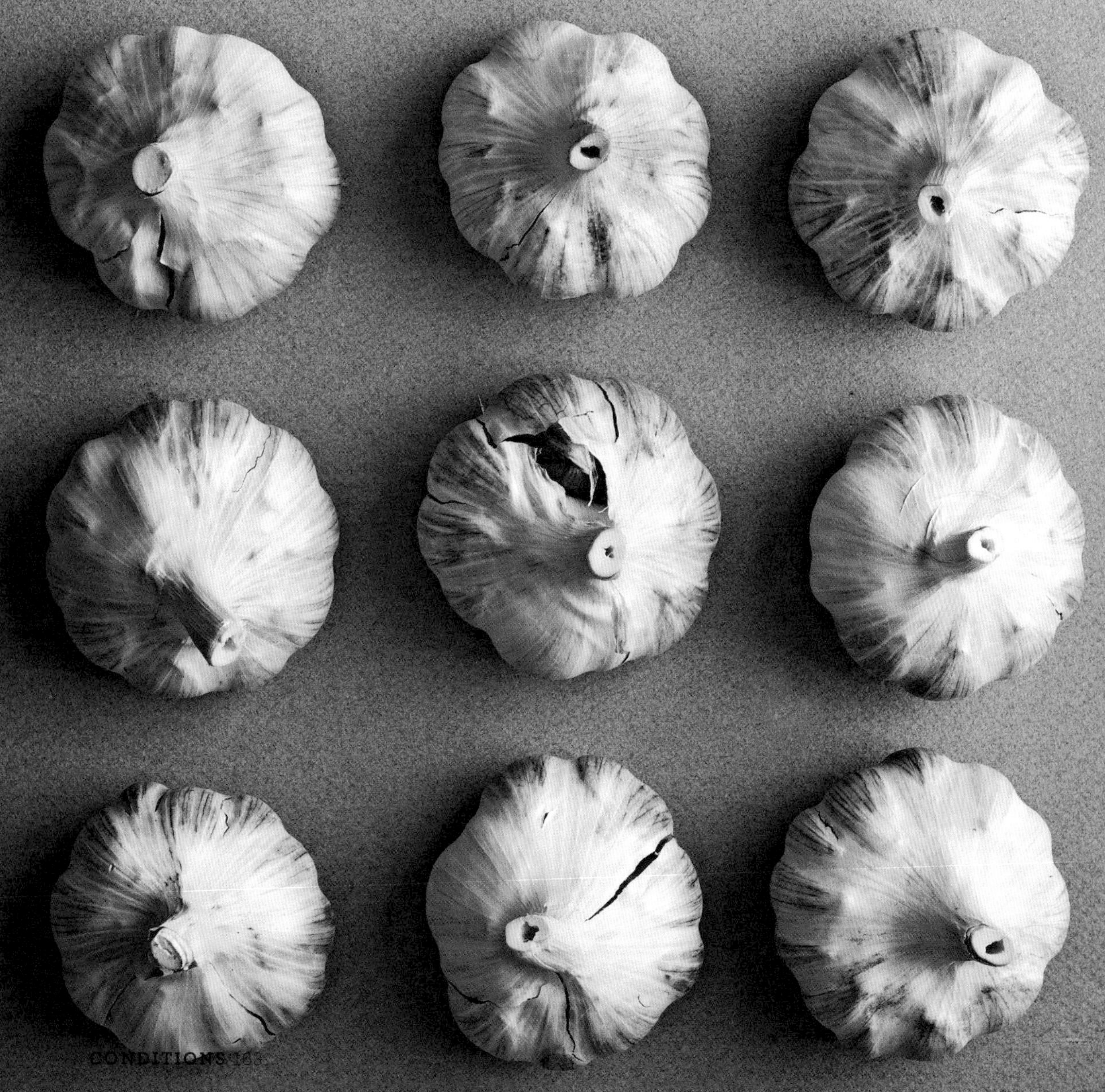

S SKIN

ACNE

Acne can be a very distressing condition—I know from experience! It is an infection of the hair follicle, during which the sebaceous glands secrete an oily substance called sebum, which lubricates the skin and hair. If sebum is over-produced, it can quickly fill the pore of the follicle and forms a blackhead. This starts to trap bacteria inside the pore that normally live happily on the surface. This causes infection, and the immune system moves in to fight it. It's the white blood cells fighting the infection that causes the redness and swelling.

Increase omega 3 to reduce inflammation

Inflammation reduction is realistically achievable through your diet. Inflammation is responsible for the redness and swelling around a spot, so reducing it will make them less severe and look better, faster. Increasing your intake of omega-3 fatty acids is one of the most powerful ways to do this, as they are the building blocks of the body's built-in inflammation management system. Omega 3 is abundant in oily fish (such as salmon, mackerel, and herring), and also in some seeds, such as flax and hemp. I recommend eating omega 3-rich foods every day if possible, trying to mix it up a little. You can also reduce your intake of oils such as vegetable, sunflower, or corn oil—olive oil is fine, though—as these are very high in omega-6 fatty acids, which can aggravate inflammation. Fat-soluble antioxidants are another important factor in reducing inflammation. They will naturally accumulate in the fatty, lower layers of the skin and offer some localized reduction in inflammation. They tend to be found in orange, yellow, and red foods.

Increase zinc to reduce infection and sebum

Infection in the hair follicle is what causes pimples to appear in the first place, so reducing infection will be of great benefit. The only real way to do this through diet is by supporting white blood cell production and activity. Zinc is one of the most important nutrients for this, as it is used by white blood cells to regulate many aspects of their function, including the rate and extent to which they move to the site of infection and defend against it. Zinc also helps regulate sebaceous gland activity, and there is some evidence to suggest that sufficient zinc intake may help reduce sebum production. Seafood, grains, nuts, and seeds are all good sources of zinc.

Regulate blood sugar

Several trials have shown a low-GI diet to be beneficial to acne sufferers. This may be because sharp rises in blood sugar release adrenaline, which stimulates the sebaceous glands to produce sebum. A diet high in fast-release carbohydrates also worsens inflammation. A low-GI diet means reducing refined carbohydrates such as white bread, white rice, white pasta, and opting for whole grain varieties instead, and also eating less of them. It also involves eating more vegetables and lean proteins. Every meal should consist of all of these elements so that it delivers its energy very slowly, and therefore does not raise blood sugar sharply.

Key ingredients:

Salmon—high in anti-inflammatory omega 3
Red peppers—packed with fat-soluble antioxidants such as flavonoids and carotenoids
Sweet potatoes, carrots & butternut squash—very rich in the fat-soluble antioxidant beta carotene
Shrimp—packed with zinc for fighting infection
Pumpkin seeds—high in zinc and essential fatty acids
Eggs—full of B vitamins, essential fatty acids, and a bit of zinc too!

Recommended recipes:

Asparagus and smoked salmon egg dippers, page 42
Heart-healthy tuna Niçoise salad, page 72
Red bell pepper and white bean dip, page 76
The beta booster, page 86
Omega pesto pasta, page 103
Sweet potato and spinach curry, page 104
Sesame soy salmon and vegetables with coconut rice, page 120
Immune-boosting jumbo shrimp curry, page 134
Salmon and jumbo shrimp skewers with citrus quinoa salad, page 142

ECZEMA

Eczema is one of the most common skin conditions of all. It is essentially an inflammatory lesion of the skin caused by an aggressive immune system reaction to something in the environment, known as a hypersensitivity reaction. This response causes patches of inflammation to appear on the skin, which will become red, raised, and incredibly itchy as the immune system goes into overdrive. Once things have calmed down a bit, the damage caused to the skin by the flare-up makes skin cells die off faster, leading to dry, flaky skin.

Increase omega 3 intake

These vital fatty acids are one of the most powerful allies in the fight against inflammation. One of the main by-products that our body manufactures when metabolizing them are prostaglandins, which help manage the inflammatory response. Some prostaglandins activate inflammation, and make it worse, while others can switch it off. The body makes whichever type it needs in response to the internal situation. However, dietary habits can also influence this picture, and different dietary fats are metabolized to form different types of prostaglandins. Omega 3 is converted into the type that quiets inflammation down, so by eating it we are helping our bodies to reduce inflammation. I'd strongly recommend eating oily fish once a day, and making good use of flaxseed oil by adding it to dips or using it for dressings, as this seed oil is also very rich in omega 3.

Reduce omega 6 intake

The other part of the omega puzzle is to reduce your intake of omega-6 fatty acids. These are vitally important fatty acids, but we only need a very small amount of them, and any excess is metabolized into a pro-inflammatory group of prostaglandins. Most of us consume more than 23 times the amount than we need a day, which is bad news for inflammation. Most omega 6 is found in vegetable oils, such as sunflower oil and margarines, which are abundant in processed, packaged foods. So, the simple message is to use olive oil for cooking, avoid margarine, and avoid processed foods like the plague.

Increase fat-soluble antioxidants

We've all heard about antioxidants and know that they're good for us. However, there are different types: some are water soluble, which means that they stay in the body for a limited time and then exit through the urine. Others are fat soluble, which means they want to move into the fatty tissues of the body, where they can be stored, including the fatty, lower layers of the skin. When we consume enough fat-soluble antioxidants, they can accumulate in these layers and have localized effects. Antioxidants are mildly anti-inflammatory, so can offer additional support in managing inflammation during a flare-up. They are found in abundance in orange, red, yellow, and pink foods.

Key ingredients:

Oily fish (salmon, mackerel, anchovies, herring)—packed with anti-inflammatory omega 3
Olive oil—low in omega 6, contains some omega 3
Red peppers—packed with fat-soluble antioxidants
Sweet potatoes, butternut squash, carrots—packed with beta carotene (the orange pigment), a very powerful fat-soluble antioxidant
Shrimp—packed with astaxanthin, a potent fat-soluble antioxidant

Recommended recipes:

Roasted butternut squash, garlic, and red lentil soup, page 56
Roasted vegetable and guacamole open sandwich, page 62
Greek pita pizza, page 70
Roast red beet wedges with avocado horseradish, page 82
Sweet potato and spinach curry, page 104
Red bell peppers stuffed with herbed goat cheese, page 106
Antioxidant salad with orange mustard dressing, page 109
Tuna steaks with sweet potato wedges and greens, page 118

PSORIASIS

Psoriasis is a relatively common skin disorder that affects the turnover of skin cells. New skin cells are formed at the very bottom layer of our skin, and gradually make their way outwards as the cells above them die and fall off. In psoriasis, this perfectly normal process goes a little haywire and moves at a much faster pace. The cause isn't completely understood, but many people now believe it is an autoimmune condition, in which our body's own immune system turns upon itself. It is thought that a type of white blood cell called a T cell moves into the dermis of the skin and releases chemical messengers called cytokines that cause local inflammatory responses, which in turn will make normal skin cells die off much more rapidly, and new cells turn over even more so. This inflammation may explain the redness and irritation that occurs at the first stage of a psoriasis flare-up. The increased skin cell turnover that follows is responsible for the characteristic silver, scaly, and flaky stage of the lesion.

Increase intake of anti-inflammatory omega 3

This in itself can greatly reduce the severity of the psoriasis, and certainly make it look a lot less red. Omega-3 fatty acids are one of the best dietary components for managing inflammation, in particular those from oily fish known as EPA and DHA, which are metabolized to form a series of communication compounds called prostaglandins that regulate the inflamatory response. There are different types of prostaglandins, but the ones made from EPA are very powerful anti-inflammatories and can reduce the redness associated with psoriasis.

Eat more orange, yellow, and red fruits and vegetables

These colors tend to be supplied by a group of compounds called carotenoids: potent fat-soluble antioxidants. We have all heard a million times that antioxidants are good for us, but not all antioxidants are equal, and they don't all do the same thing. They can be placed into two distinct categories. Some are water soluble and will not be stored in the body. They deliver their actions in our general circulation for a limited period of time, then get excreted through the urine. Other antioxidants, like the carotenoids, are fat soluble. This means they naturally migrate into fatty tissues like the subcutaneous layer of the skin, where they can accumulate and be available on standby to deliver their actions locally. Their anti-inflammatory activity can help to reduce the redness and swelling.

Eat quercetin-rich foods
Quercetin is a phytochemical compound that is often thought of as being a natural antihistamine. This is indeed true, but quercetin is also starting to show some promise in the treatment of skin problems because it inhibits the activity of an enzyme called phospholipase, which removes a fatty acid called arachidonic acid from our cells. Arachidonic acid is then converted into a compound that stimulates inflammation. Reducing the liberation of this fatty acid adds to the reduction in inflammation and redness.

Increase your B vitamin intake
These commonly deficient nutrients are vital for the overall health of the skin. They regulate many responses, including regulating the turnaround of skin cells and microcirculation to the outer layers of the skin, which enhances skin tone.

Key ingredients:
Mackerel—packed with anti-inflammatory omega 3
Sweet potatoes, butternut squash, carrots—packed with carotenoids, the potent fat-soluble antioxidants
Red peppers—another rich source of fat-soluble antioxidants
Onions, leeks, garlic—packed with quercetin
Avocado—rich in fat-soluble antioxidant vitamin E
Brown rice—rich in B vitamins
Shrimp—rich in zinc and selenium

Recommended recipes:
The beta booster, page 86
Skin-boosting guacamole, page 92
Red bell peppers stuffed with herbed goat cheese, page 106
Baked sweet potatoes with omega hummus, page 110
Roasted bell peppers with white bean mash, page 116
Broiled salmon with spinach and spiced carrot mash, page 138

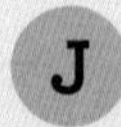

JOINTS & BONES

ARTHRITIS (RHEUMATOID)

Rheumatoid arthritis is an autoimmune condition in which our body's immune system attacks the lining of the joint, causing it to become inflamed. This can lead to structures within the joint being destroyed, and even to joint disfigurement. Although the root cause is the dysfunction in the immune system, managing inflammation is one of the key areas in which diet can offer the most help. It won't offer an alternative to regular medical treatment, but will go a long way to improving your self-management of the condition.

Increase omega 3 intake to manage inflammation
Increasing our consumption of omega-3 fatty acids, the amazing "good fats" we hear so much about, can help with inflammation. These are the building blocks for a group of communication chemicals that reduce the inflammatory response. There are a few different types of omega 3, which are all important in managing inflammation effectively. I recommend eating more oily fish, as they contain the highest levels and broadest spectrum of omega 3. The British Dietetic Association advises 2–3 portions per week, but if you can eat more, great! If you are vegetarian, eating flax seeds and flaxseed oil goes a long way toward getting the balance right, and you can consider supplements. Antioxidants can also help, as these "buzz" compounds can reduce some of the free radicals released during the inflammatory response, which can exacerbate it.

Key ingredients:
Oily fish (salmon, herring, mackerel, sardines, anchovies)—rich in the all-important omega 3
Pineapple—contains the anti-inflammatory enzyme bromelain
Turmeric—contains curcuminoids, the anti-inflammatory colour pigments
Celery—contains 3-n-butylphthalide, a natural painkiller
Brightly colored fruits and vegetables—packed with antioxidants

Recommended recipes:
Asparagus and smoked salmon egg dippers, page 42
Thai fish soup, page 50
Gazpacho, page 58
The beta booster, page 86
Sweet potato and spinach curry, page 104
Sesame soy salmon and vegetables with coconut rice, page 120
Salmon and jumbo shrimp skewers with citrus quinoa salad, page 142

BURSITIS

Bursitis is an inflammation of the bursae, the fluid-filled sacks in the joints that provide cushioning where bone, muscle, and tendons rub against each other, allowing flawless, smooth movement. The inflammation can arise from manual labor, demanding exercise regimes or injury to the joint. Bursitis is often painful, and nothing will replace some heavy-duty anti-inflammatories from your doctor. However, your diet can certainly enhance their action, and really help you on your road to recovery.

Increase omega 3 intake to manage inflammation

The stars of the show once again are the omega-3 fatty acids, the building blocks for a group of communication chemicals in the body that reduce the inflammatory response. There are a few different types of omega 3, which are all important. I recommend eating more oily fish, as they contain the highest levels and broadest spectrum of omega 3. If you are vegetarian, eating flax seeds and flaxseed oil goes a long way toward getting the balance right, and you can consider supplements. Turmeric has also been studied for its anti-inflammatory activity. A group of compounds called curcuminoids (which give its bright orange color), block certain aspects of the inflammatory response.

Key ingredients:

Oily fish (salmon, mackerel, herring)—packed with anti-inflammatory omega 3
Olive oil in place of other cooking oils—increases omega 3 and reduces omega 6, a fat that can worsen inflammation if consumed to excess
Turmeric—anti-inflammatory
Brightly colored fruits and vegetables—high antioxidant, which assists in reducing inflammation

Recommended recipes:

Purple power salad, page 78
Omega pesto pasta, page 103
Sweet potato and spinach curry, page 104
Baked sweet potatoes with omega hummus, page 110
Tuna steaks with sweet potato wedges and greens, page 118
Broiled salmon with spinach and spiced carrot mash, page 138

OSTEOPOROSIS

Osteoporosis is caused by a loss of bone density, which increases the risk of fractures. Starting from around the age of 35, bone density begins to decline, and certain lifestyle choices can increase this process. Sedentary living, being underweight, and drinking too much can make this situation much worse. Menopausal women are also at greater risk of osteoporosis, as estrogen is involved in maintaining bone density, and when it begins to drop, this will have negative repercussions for the skeleton.

Increase vitamin D intake

Vitamin D is one of the biggest missing components in bone health. Although calcium is the structural material that the bones are made of, without the auxiliary nutrients that help it do its thing, it is pretty much useless. Vitamin D is vital for getting adequate amounts of calcium into the bloodstream. Our primary source of vitamin D is the conversion of cholesterol into vitamin D precursors when the skin is exposed to UV radiation in sunlight. Depending on where you live, this can be a problem, so it's essential that we also look for as many dietary sources of vitamin D as possible.

Increase magnesium-rich foods

Magnesium is another forgotten nutrient that is vital for a healthy skeleton. Magnesium plays a vital role in the way in which calcium is metabolized and utilized. It is required for the proper formation of calcitriol, the active form of vitamin D responsible for increasing calcium levels in the blood. Adequate magnesium intake also reduces the release of parathyroid hormone (PTH), a hormone which causes an increased release of calcium from the skeleton, something we desperately need to avoid in osteoporosis.

Increase phyto-oestrogen-rich foods

For menopausal women, consuming foods rich in phytoestrogens may help to reduce bone density loss by providing estrogen-like compounds to the body.

Up the oily fish

We now know that one particular omega-3 fatty acid called DHA is involved in maintaining stronger bones. While it is possible to get plant-derived DHA in supplement form, oily fish is a quick and simple way of getting adequate amounts in each day.

Key ingredients:

Eggs—rich in vitamin D
Feta & goat cheese—rich in calcium and vitamin D
Kale—dense source of magnesium
Miso paste—very rich source of phytoestrogens
Salmon—packed with the omega-3 fatty acid, DHA
Mackerel, anchovies—high in vitamin D and DHA

Recommended recipes:

Spinach and feta scramble, page 31
Calming green soup, page 52
Heart-healthy tuna Niçoise salad, page 72
Stress-free smoked mackerel pâté, page 92

RICKETS & OSTEOMALACIA

Rickets is a serious softening of the bones that occurs in children, while osteomalacia is a similar softening of the bones that manifests in adults. Both conditions are linked to low levels of calcium caused by a lack of vitamin D, which regulates how the body uses calcium. A lack of it can drastically affect the amount of calcium we absorb from our food. These conditions used to be a thing of the past, but in recent years have started to appear again. There are several factors thought to be responsible for this, but a combination of poor diet and lack of sunshine could both be contributing factors.

Increase vitamin D intake
Our primary source of vitamin D is the conversion of cholesterol into vitamin D precursors when the skin is exposed to UV radiation—in other words, the sun! However, there are a few good dietary sources of vitamin D that can help to make up for the deficit that some of us experience.

Increase high-quality calcium intake
Many people with these conditions look toward calcium supplements to remedy their drop in calcium. This may be helpful in certain circumstances, under the guidance of a practitioner, but often the calcium in these supplements is of a poor quality and isn't very well absorbed. There have also recently been links between calcium supplementation (without the correct guidance) and heart and kidney problems. Therefore, I feel it is best to focus upon dietary sources. This doesn't mean guzzling pints and pints of milk, though, as that will bring its own set of problems. Dairy produce can be a good source of dietary calcium, but there are so many more. Many green vegetables, nuts, seeds, beans, even fish, are useful sources. The wider the variety you consume the better, in my opinion.

Key ingredients:
Mackerel, salmon—packed with vitamin D
Anchovies—vitamin D and packed with calcium
Eggs—vitamin D and calcium
Almonds—a great source of easy-to-absorb calcium
Feta & goat cheese, yogurt—calcium-rich, easy to digest

Recommended recipes:
Spinach and feta scramble, page 31
Calming green soup, page 52
Red bell peppers stuffed with herbed goat cheese, page 106
Red beet, red onion, and goat cheese tart, page 130

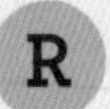 RESPIRATORY SYSTEM

ASTHMA

Asthma is a localized inflammation of the bronchioles (tiny passageways in the lungs) caused by sensitivity to environmental triggers such as dust, environmental pollutants, and dust mites. When we are exposed to the trigger stimuli, the immune system responds, causing inflammation. This rapidly narrows the airways and causes difficulty in breathing. Now, I don't believe food is often a cause, but I do believe that manipulating our intake of certain foods and nutrients will improve things.

Increase omega 3 to reduce inflammation
Diet can go a long way to reducing inflammation. Some of the most powerful regulators of inflammation are the omega-3 fatty acids, abundant in oily fish, olive oil, walnuts, flax seeds, and flax oil.

Eat Mediterranean food
Some studies have associated a Mediterranean diet with a lower incidence of asthma symptoms. This makes perfect sense, as it's rich in fruit, vegetables, olive oil, and fish, and low in saturated fats and refined carbohydrates. It's perfect for controlling inflammation with its abundance of omega 3, antioxidants, and vitamins.

Increase vitamin C to reduce histamine
The chemical histamine, which is released by some white blood cells during an allergic response, is the catalyst that triggers the inflammation. It causes the airways to swell and constrict, and therefore the breathlessness during an attack. Onions contain quercetin, which reduces the amount of histamine released. Foods high in vitamin C, such as red peppers, citrus fruit, and spinach, also reduce histamine release.

Key ingredients:
Oily fish (salmon, anchovies, herring, mackerel)—high in anti-inflammatory omega 3
Flax seeds & oil—high in anti-inflammatory omega 3
Onions—high in antihistamine quercetin
Red peppers, citrus, spinach—rich in vitamin C
Horseradish—believed by some to widen the airways

Recommended recipes:
Heart-healthy tuna Niçoise salad, page 72
Omega pesto pasta, page 103
Roasted bell peppers with white bean mash, page 116
Sesame soy salmon and vegetables with coconut rice, page 120
Baked salmon with herbed omega crust, page 132
Mackerel marinated with red beets and horseradish, page 140

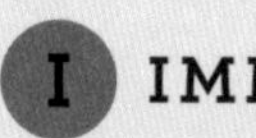

IMMUNE SYSTEM

COLDS & FLU

There is no "cure" for the common cold, but I firmly believe there is a lot we can do to make ourselves feel better by reducing symptoms, and also by improving our body's way of dealing with such infections. Cold and flu viruses attack the upper respiratory tract, such as the nose and throat. When they get into these tissues and start causing mischief, our immune system responds by sending an army of white blood cells to the area to kill the virus. It is the immune system trying to control the infection that gives us the symptoms associated with cold and flu.

Improve your immune system

This is a contentious subject, but some foods have shown some positive results in several types of study. Shiitake mushrooms and goji berries contain unique, active sugars called polysaccharides. These have demonstrated some interesting effects on our immune system, and shiitake polysaccharides have been shown to increase the production of white blood cells. The more we can produce during an infection, the better the position we are to deal with it effectively. Our body does increase production of white cells during an infection, but shiitake mushrooms may step this up even further. Goji-berry polysaccharides have shown similar activity, but to date the research is more limited. More needs to be done, but it looks as though they might increase the white blood cell count too. Zinc can also enhance immune response. White blood cells use zinc to code DNA, which works as an internal control mechanism for the cell, helping it respond to invaders and pathogens. Many trials have shown that increasing our intake of zinc-rich foods can improve resilience to infections, and also the time it takes to recover from infection.

Eat more garlic

Garlic is well known as a potent antiviral. Unlike most compounds, which are removed through the kidneys and bowel, the essential oils in garlic cannot be removed this way, and are instead removed through the breath. As they move through the respiratory tract, they can pick off the bugs and viruses lurking there, waiting to cause trouble.

Reduce inflammation

Tissues in the upper respiratory tract become inflamed during colds and flu while the immune system is dealing with the infection. Reducing this inflammation goes a long way toward making us feel more human again. One of my favorite ingredients when I have a touch of the dreaded man flu is the old faithful ginger! This contains a very powerful anti-inflammatory ingredient, part of the chemistry that gives ginger its powerful spicy aroma, which works by blocking the manufacture of compounds that activate inflammation. Omega-3 fatty acids in foods such as oily fish and flax seeds are also of great value in helping the body make its own natural anti-inflammatory compounds.

Key ingredients:
Shiitake mushrooms—powerful polysaccharides support immune function
Garlic—antiviral
Ginger—anti-inflammatory
Chili peppers—decongestant
Goji berries—likely to support immune function
Sweet potatoes—mild anti-inflammatory
Water, lots of it—beats dehydration from fever that often accompanies colds and flu
Shrimp—packed with zinc
Coconut—contains lauric acid, a natural antiviral

Recommended recipes:
Spinach, tomato, and shiitake mushrooms on toast, page 40
The famous flu fighter, page 48
Holy shiitake, page 68
Immune-boosting jumbo shrimp curry, page 134

M METABOLIC SYSTEM

DIABETES (TYPE 2)

Type 2 is the most common kind of diabetes, and is related to diet and lifestyle. It occurs when our body's blood-sugar management system starts to fail. When the energy from food is released into the bloodstream in the form of glucose, a hormone called insulin is produced to take the sugar out of the blood into our cells to be turned into energy. Blood sugar also needs to stay low for the health of many tissues. However, many of us are eating too many foods that cause huge rises in blood sugar levels, such as white bread, white rice, white pasta, and sugary snacks and drinks. These release their glucose very quickly, and the body's response is a massive release of insulin to get it out of the bloodstream as rapidly as it can. This is fine occasionally, but if we do it regularly the blood cells start ignoring what the insulin is saying to them, and as a result are much less inclined to take up the excess sugar. So our blood sugar stays high, and this causes many problems. This is the beginning of type 2 diabetes, and is known as "insulin resistance."

Eat a low-GI diet

This means eating food that releases its energy gradually, thus avoiding blood-sugar spikes. The first step is to ditch refined carbohydrates forever—foods like white bread, white rice, white pasta, chocolate bars, sugary snacks, and drinks. They are full of very simple sugars that take virtually no digestive effort to release, and can therefore enter the bloodstream rapidly, sending blood sugar levels sky high. Opt for whole grain versions of bread and pasta, and save treats like chocolate bars for very, very special occasions. It's even more beneficial to reduce carbohydrate intake right across the board. Eat much smaller portions of carbohydrates than you have been used to. Next, make sure you eat a good-quality, complex carbohydrate (such as whole grains, brown rice or quinoa) and a good-quality protein at each meal, and preferably a high-quality fat, too. Meals composed like this take longer to digest and release their energy slowly and consistently, without those problematic blood sugar spikes.

Increase omega 3 intake

Recent research has suggested that omega-3 fatty acids in our cells can make insulin receptors more sensitive to insulin signalling. These receptors are built into the walls of our cells. Fatty acids from food form part of the structure of these walls and receptors alike. Different fatty acids will affect the way in which the cell membrane wall and the receptors work. Omega-3 fatty acids often show improved functioning of many facets of cell membranes and receptors.

A bit of chocolate may do you good

Some studies have shown that regular consumption of a little bit of dark chocolate can improve insulin responsiveness. It is believed the flavanol compounds in chocolate are responsible for this. The exact way these compounds deliver this effect remains unclear, but I'm sure it will come as good news for some! Try to find the lowest sugar, highest quality dark chocolate possible.

Key ingredients:

Low-GI grains (such as brown rice, quinoa, bulgur wheat)—much lower GI than their refined relatives
Lean proteins such as oily fish, tofu, eggs—these are masters at controlling the glycemic response to food, and oily fish are packed with omega 3
Artichokes—Contain inulin, which stabilizes blood sugar levels
Cinnamon—May play a role in blood sugar balance

Recommended recipes:

Spinach and feta scramble, page 31
Kick-starter kedgeree, page 44
Tomato and lentil soup, page 54
Creamy egg on rye with wild arugula, page 64
Smoked trout and quinoa salad, page 115
Tuna steaks with sweet potato wedges and greens, page 118

N MENTAL HEALTH & NERVOUS SYSTEM

ANXIETY

Anxiety, or Generalized Anxiety Disorder (GAD), is a very common problem, and increasingly more so. Symptoms can include palpitations, sweating, shortness of breath and hyperventilating, dizziness, racing mind, and feelings of fear or intense worry. Now, diet will never be your saving grace, but good dietary choices will certainly help. If you have been prescribed medication for your anxiety, it's important not to stop taking it. The dietary strategies below will work beautifully side by side with it. Safe and delicious!

Stabilize blood-sugar levels

One of the quickest ways to send your mind and mood reeling is to eat fast-release carbohydrates like sugary drinks and snacks and white bread. These foods cause a sugar rush and a surge of adrenaline that can make us feel manic and edgy. Adrenaline is to anxiety what kerosene is to a bonfire! On top of that, the body has to deal with this sugar at a rapid pace, and what goes up must come down, so we are left in a slump. This causes low moods and mental fog. A low-GI diet will keep blood sugar levels at a steady and consistent level, keeping moods stable and preventing mood swings and brain fog. To follow a low-GI diet, eliminate refined carbohydrates such as sugary snacks and drinks, white bread, white rice, and white pasta. Choose whole grain breads, pasta, and rice, and always include a high-quality protein with each meal. Make sure you include plenty of good fats (see below). This will mean that you will be eating foods that release their sugar more slowly and don't upset blood sugar balance. Most of the dishes in this book are low GI.

Increase omega 3 intake

Omega-3 fatty acids have been widely studied for their effect on mental functioning, including anxiety, and many studies have shown a notable improvement in symptoms. The exact way this works isn't fully understood, but we do know that it helps with signalling and communication within the brain. It is also believed that omega 3 can aid the release of "feel-good" chemicals in the brain, helping to lift the mood. Omega 3 can also control inflammation by causing the body to manufacture its own natural anti-inflammatory compounds. It is richest in oily fish, which contain the full spectrum of omega-3 fatty acids needed for brain health. Include as much salmon, mackerel, herring, and fresh tuna in your diet as possible. If you are vegetarian, you can increase your intake of seeds such as flax seeds, but you may need to consider using supplements.

Increase magnesium-rich foods

Many clinical trials have shown that magnesium is an important factor in anxiety. It is involved in physical relaxation, including the relaxation of skeletal muscles, and also in regulating many enzyme systems in the body. Whether magnesium will affect the nervous system directly is unclear, but by aiding muscle relaxation, it will certainly help us to feel more relaxed. Magnesium-rich foods include green, leafy vegetables, nuts, and seeds.

Key ingredients:

Low-GI grains (such as brown rice, quinoa, bulgur wheat)—much lower GI than their refined relatives
Oily fish (salmon, mackerel, herring, tuna, anchovies)—packed with omega-3 fatty acids
Sunflower seeds—rich source of magnesium
Kale & greens—rich in magnesium
Dark chocolate/cacao powder—very rich source of magnesium

Recommended recipes:

Spinach and feta scramble, page 31
Thai fish soup, page 50
Stir-fried satay greens, page 75
Garlicky white beans with kale and Parmesan, page 84
Baked sweet potatoes with omega hummus, page 110
Sesame soy salmon and vegetables with coconut rice, page 120
Salmon and jumbo shrimp skewers with citrus quinoa salad, page 142
Chocolate morning smoothie, page 155

DEPRESSION

Depression is greatly misunderstood by those who have never experienced it, and is sometimes viewed as something we can "snap out of." But there is now a lot of evidence to show that it is as much biochemical as psychological, and most likely an interaction between the two. We don't fully understand what occurs in the brain during depression, but it's likely that there are biochemical changes, and that environmental, physical and emotional factors may cause this disturbance.

Eat protein and complex carbohydrates together at each meal

Keeping our blood sugar levels stable is important for all brain and mood-related issues. Fluctuations in blood sugar can affect our concentration, moods, focus, ability to think clearly, not to mention our energy levels. By combining protein with complex carbohydrates (such as whole grains, brown rice, or quinoa), we will digest much more slowly, and energy will be released more steadily and consistently. This will drip-feed the blood sugar, keeping levels stable. Proteins also contain an amino acid called tryptophan. This gets converted in the brain to a substance called serotonin, the "feel-good" chemical in our brain. This amino acid needs a bit of help getting across what is called the "blood brain barrier," to enter the brain and get turned into serotonin. A subtle lift in insulin (the chemical released when we eat carbohydrate-rich foods that tells our cells to absorb the sugars from our bloodstream) can help with this. Eating a protein-rich food with a complex carbohydrate will supply a good source of tryptophan and give a little increase in insulin to take it where it needs to go.

Eat small, regular meals
Eating smaller meals every 2–3 hours may be better than sitting down to three big meals a day, as it will help regulate blood sugar levels.

Eat more oily fish
Oily fish is unique in containing the full spectrum of types of omega-3 fatty acids, including EPA, which is not found in plant sources. EPA has been studied broadly in the context of depression, and has delivered some encouraging results, including mood elevation and an increased ability to focus. Similar effects have not been found in omega 3 from plant sources. Oily fish such as salmon and mackerel are the best sources of EPA.

Increase B vitamin intake
These essential nutrients are involved in many aspects of brain function, including the production of neurotransmitters in the brain. Several studies have linked low levels of B12 with symptoms of depression, and increased B12 with a better response to treatments for depression. Eat plenty of whole grains like brown rice, quinoa, bulgur wheat, mushrooms, asparagus, eggs, and yeast extract.

Key ingredients:
Oily fish (salmon, mackerel, herring)—rich sources of the omega-3 fatty acid EPA
Brown rice—rich in B vitamins
Eggs—rich in B vitamins, including B12

Recommended recipes:
Herbed Mediterranean frittata, page 36
Kick-starter kedgeree, page 44
Thai fish soup, page 50
Sesame soy salmon and vegetables with coconut rice, page 120
Salmon and jumbo shrimp skewers with citrus quinoa salad, page 142

INSOMNIA

A good 6–8 hours of sleep every night is essential for the proper repair and maintenance of the body. Any less than this on a regular basis can be very bad for our health, but there is no single factor that causes insomnia. It can be related to worry, excessive caffeine or alcohol intake, or a sign of a more serious underlying illness. Persistent insomnia should be referred to your doctor, but occasional bouts may respond very well to food.

Increase tryptophan-rich foods
Tryptophan is a naturally occurring amino acid that is the chemical building block of a neurotransmitter called melatonin. This chemical sets sleep patterns, and can help us to get a deeper, longer sleep. Dietary sources of tryptophan, when consumed with a complex carbohydrate (which helps it get to where it is needed, the brain), can help us get off to sleep and keep us there.

Increase magnesium intake
Magnesium is a potent muscle relaxant. Consuming extra magnesium in the evening can help us physically relax more and drift off to sleep a little easier.

Avoid refined carbohydrates
These are things like white bread, white rice, white pasta, sugary snacks and drinks. This type of refined carbohydrate can send our blood sugar levels soaring, causing episodes of irritability and a racing mind, and will stop us from switching off. Their complex carbohydrate cousins, however, are helpful because they help with the absorption of tryptophan.

Key ingredients:
Bananas—rich in tryptophan
Cherries—rich in melatonin, a sleep-inducing hormone
Green leafy vegetables—packed with magnesium
Tuna—rich source of tryptophan
Low-GI grains (such as brown rice, quinoa, bulgur wheat)—much lower GI than their refined relatives

Recommended recipes:
Banana-peanut oat bars, page 98
Kale and potato salad with peanut chili sauce, page 114
Tuna steaks with sweet potato wedges and greens, page 118
Goodnight spiced cherry crumble, page 146

MIGRAINE

Migraines cause misery to many people, but are poorly understood. We do know that blood vessels in the head and neck contract, then dilate rapidly in response to a stimulus of some kind. The constriction is believed to be responsible for much of the visual disturbance experienced by migraine sufferers, and the sudden dilation that follows causes the headache. For some people, this can be linked to triggers such as red wine and chocolate, or even just low blood sugar. For others, there may be no easily definable link to speak of.

Increase magnesium intake

It is thought that low concentrations of magnesium in the brain is a trend in migraine sufferers, and increased magnesium intake has a good track record, anecdotally at least, in the management of the condition. Magnesium is involved in energy production, muscle relaxation, correct functioning of the nervous system, and over 1,000 other biological reactions, so what has been reported by sufferers is certainly plausible. The best food sources of magnesium are greens. Magnesium is to plants what iron is to humans, and is a key component of chlorophyll, the green color pigment in plants. If it's green, it's packed with magnesium.

Increase omega 3 intake

There is evidence to suggest that reducing inflammation in the body can be beneficial in cases of migraine. One of the best ways to do this through diet is to increase your intake of omega-3 fatty acids, in particular EPA and DHA from oily fish. These are metabolized in the body to form our own natural, built-in anti-inflamatory compounds, the prostaglandins.

Key ingredients:

Leafy greens such as kale—packed with magnesium
Salmon and other oily fish (mackerel, herring)—rich source of EPA and DHA

Recommended recipes:

Asparagus and smoked salmon egg dippers, page 42
Kale and potato salad with peanut chili sauce, page 114

STRESS

Some types of stress can be useful, but what makes frequent and regular stress so bad is the surge of hormones, such as adrenaline and cortisol, which increase blood pressure and make the heart beat harder and faster to get more oxygen to our tissues and make us react faster and work harder. They also cause our body to secrete insulin to make our cells take up more sugar so that they can perform better to get us out of the dangerous situation. All of these responses are vital, and when they only happen every now and again the hormones are quickly broken down and our physiology returns to normal. However, when we are in a regular state of stress, this response happens frequently, which can raise our blood pressure significantly and increase our risk of heart disease. We also start to accumulate the stress hormone cortisol. When this happens, we start to make fewer and fewer white blood cells, which affects our immune system. Our digestive system is impaired and the absorption of nutrients is reduced, which affects our nutritional status and has a knock-on effect on our health. The nervous system and adrenal glands take a beating too, which can lead to anxiety, angry outbursts, exhaustion, and even breakdown. Now, of course food won't remo,ve the source of stress, but what you eat can certainly help ease the physiological implications.

Blood sugar management

Fluctuations in blood sugar can drastically affect our mood and have a major impact on the way we respond to stressful stimuli. When our blood sugar shoots up, we can feel as though we can take on anything, and are also less prone to reacting negatively to stressful situations. When our blood sugar dips too low, however, we can feel lethargic, depressed, anxious, and moody, and the smallest of stressors can send us over the edge. By focusing on low-GI ingredients that release their energy slowly, we can keep levels much more stable. These types of foods include whole grains, lean proteins, healthy fats, and, of course, fresh, wholesome fruits and vegetables. The way we compose meals can help stabilize blood sugar even further: try to ensure that each meal contains a complex carbohydrate such as brown rice, wholemeal bread or quinoa; a lean protein such as fish, poultry or lean dairy produce; some healthy fats such as olive olive or avocado; and some fruit or vegetables. When meals are composed in this way they release their energy much more slowly.

Increase omega 3 intake

For anxiety, mood swings, anger, depression, or even mental burnout, omega 3 should have pride of place in your armory. There is a lot of research to support the use of omega 3 in these situations. Adequate omega 3 can improve the way our nervous system uses our "feel-good" brain chemicals, and can reduce the negative impact that prolonged stress can have on the nervous system. When we are under prolonged stress and begin to accumulate cortisol and insulin spikes from adrenaline surges, we create more inflammation in the body, which, over time, can increase our risk of many chronic diseases. Omega 3 helps the body manufacture its own built-in anti-inflammatory compounds.

Increase B vitamin intake

The B vitamins are a vital component in the dietary management of stress. They are involved in supporting healthy adrenal glands and a healthy nervous system. During bouts of stress, they are used up very quickly, and many of us are deficient in them as a result. Couple this with the generally poor intake of B vitamins in the western diet anyway, and you can see how rapidly deficiency arises.

Increase zinc intake
This vital mineral is important in the management of stress in two distinct ways. Firstly, prolonged stress negatively affects the immune system, and many people going through stressful periods find they pick up all manner of colds and infections. Zinc supports our immune system because it helps our white blood cells code genetic material that helps regulate the way in which they respond to bugs. That is why zinc is so effective when we have a cold. The second reason that zinc is useful is that it is involved in regulating the effect of serotonin, our brain's "feel-good" chemical. There have been numerous links between low zinc status and depression and low mood.

Eat more magnesium-rich foods
Magnesium is a big factor in stress, as it can help us feel more relaxed. Magnesium works in our muscles to help muscle fibers relax, physically making us less tense and wound up.

Key ingredients:
Brown rice, bulgur wheat, oats—high in B vitamins
Salmon—rich in omega 3
Green leafy vegetables, such as kale—all greens are very high in magnesium
Shrimp—packed with zinc and some omega 3
Pumpkin seeds—packed with zinc

Recommended recipes:
Creamy egg on rye with wild arugula, page 64
Stir-fried satay greens, page 75
Stress-free smoked mackerel pâté, page 92
Banana-peanut oat bars, page 98
Baked salmon with herbed omega crust, page 132
Salmon and jumbo shrimp skewers with citrus quinoa salad, page 142

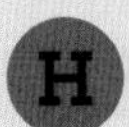

HEART & CIRCULATION

HIGH CHOLESTEROL

Cholesterol is a vital substance. All our steroidal hormones, such as estrogen and testosterone, are made from it. It is a major structural component of our cell membranes, and a precursor for vitamin D. However, too much of it can be a problem. Another issue is whether the balance between the two types, HDL and LDL, is favorable. Cholesterol has become a focal point for many patients and practitioners; it is one of the key indicators of heart disease risk, and many people are taking some kind of cholesterol-lowering drugs. There are many factors that can affect cholesterol levels, but one of the most profound is diet—thankfully, the one we have most control over on a day-to-day basis.

Achieve the right levels of good and bad fat
For the last few decades, we've all had it drummed into us that we should be cutting the amount of fat we eat to look after our hearts. However, dietary fats are a vital component of good health, and eating the right fats in the right amounts can actually improve our cholesterol levels by increasing high-density lipoprotein (HDL, the carrier protein that transports cholesterol away from the cells and back to the liver for breakdown and removal), and reducing our levels of low-density lipoprotein (LDL, the carrier protein that transports freshly made cholesterol from the liver, out into the body tissues). When we reduce our total intake of fat, we reduce our LDL, and our HDL too, which is equally as bad for the heart in the long run.

The other part of the problem is that some products that have been touted as containing "heart-healthy unsaturated fats" are actually high in a new and much nastier kind: trans fats. These have been chemically altered to change the physical properties of the products they're in, and can also occur as a byproduct of processing techniques. Many vegetable-fat spreads, for example, are made from sunflower oil, which is liquid at room temperature. To get it to behave more like butter, its chemical structure is literally inverted, creating trans fats: great for the food manufacturers, but not the body. Trans fats can rapidly reduce HDL levels, and send up LDL. They can also trigger localized inflammation, which is a major factor in the onset of heart disease. Instead, our focus should be on increasing our intake of the good fats, and avoiding the bad ones. The good fats are the essential fatty acids, omega 3, 6, and 9. Omega 3 should dominate, as these have the best effect upon cholesterol levels, reducing LDL and elevating HDL. There are also other benefits for the heart, such as reduction of clotting risk, and blood pressure. Use olive oil for cooking and coconut oils to reduce trans fat formation. Olive oil is also particularly rich in oleic acid, the omega-9 fatty acid that has been shown to have a positive impact on cholesterol levels.

Be carbohydrate-smart

The other result of the exodus away from fatty foods is that we are now consuming a lot more carbohydrates. This needn't be a disaster, but unfortunately we're eating too many refined carbohydrates such as white bread, white rice, white pasta, sugar, sweets, and chocolate. These are very rapidly digested and release their sugars very quickly, causing a huge surge in blood sugar. These can have very serious consequences, so our bodies have very effective mechanisms to manage them. The first part is the secretion of the hormone insulin, which tells our cells to take in sugar more rapidly, so it can be used for energy. It is a very effective, very rapid system. However, only a fixed amount of glucose can enter the cells at one time. When the capacity to take in glucose is exceeded (which is very possible after eating fast-release carbohydrates), another mechanism kicks in to get blood sugar levels down, in which excess sugar can be converted into (bad) LDL. Hey presto, our LDL levels go up. However, good-quality carbohydrates such as those you find in whole grains, legumes, and lightly cooked vegetables will have a stabilizing effect on blood sugar, and avoid all this. They're also great sources of B vitamins and minerals, so they should really be your only carbohydrate choices.

Eat more fiber

As well as keeping us regular, fiber is also important for keeping cholesterol in check. Cholesterol is made in the liver. Some of it enters our bloodstream directly, and some of it is carried away from the liver through the gall bladder, then into the digestive tract, from where it is absorbed into the blood. Certain fibers, especially soluble fibers, such as those found in apples, some seeds, and legumes, physically bind to cholesterol in the digestive tract, and carry it away through the bowel. Soluble fiber binds to this free cholesterol in the digestive tract, preventing it from being absorbed.

Key ingredients:

Apples—rich in pectin, a highly effective soluble fiber
Shiitake mushrooms—contain eritadenine, which has been shown to raise HDL and lower LDL
Pumpkin seeds—high in beta-sitosterol
Salmon, anchovies, tuna—rich in omega 3
Mackerel—rich in omega 3
Oats, bulgur wheat—high in beta glucan, an effective soluble fiber
Dates—high in beta glucan

Recommended recipes:

Holy shiitake, page 68
Apple and cinnamon oat squares, page 94
Vegetable crumble with cheesy oat topping, page 123
Chickpea and sweet potato beta bake, page 126
Baked eggplant with tomato and lentil stuffing, page 129
Baked salmon with herbed omega crust, page 132
Oat-crusted tuna steak with asparagus purée, page 136
Baked spiced apple wedges with heart-healthy compote, page 150

HIGH BLOOD PRESSURE

High blood pressure, or hypertension, is one of the biggest risk factors for heart disease, heart attack, and strokes. Pressure in the blood vessels is regulated by the contraction and relaxation of their muscular walls in response to the physical demands on the body. There are many factors that can affect it, including physical activity and movement, stress, diet, and age. Dietary factors can cause an increase in both contraction and relaxation of the vessels, and also affect the flexibility and responsiveness of the muscle. The higher the pressure, the greater the friction against the inner skin that lines the vessels, which can cause damage. When this happens, the vessel lining bleeds and clots can form, which can lead to serious problems.

Reduce salt intake

You've heard it a million times before, but reducing salt is necessary. To be more precise, it's sodium that we need to reduce. Many dietary minerals take the form of salts, all of which are vital for our health, including sodium; the problem is dosage. Sodium reduces urinary output, which helps the body retain water. When this happens, the watery part of our blood, the serum, gets larger, and blood pressure rises. Sodium is also vasoconstrictive: it causes the vessel walls to constrict and narrow, adding to the pressure. However, we do need some salt, and thankfully there are some on the market that are very low in sodium and high in other minerals. They give a salty flavor but don't impact so much on blood pressure, and make a perfect alternative to table salt. The other part of the picture is the hidden salt in many ready-made foods, packaged meals, and sandwiches. This shows the importance of eating fresh food, and cooking your own food as much as you can.

Increase potassium levels

Potassium is almost like the antidote for too much sodium, and reduces its effects in many ways. Research has shown that higher intakes of potassium are linked with lower blood pressure and related complications.

It isn't clear exactly how this works, but there are several theories. Potassium may reduce the responsiveness of blood vessels to the hormonal signalling that may increase blood pressure. It may also display the opposite effect on blood vessels—in other words, relaxing them.

Reduce caffeine
I don't often talk about reducing or cutting things out, but in the case of hypertension, reducing your intake of strong caffeine in filter coffee and energy drinks can be vitally important. The caffeine can have a double-whammy effect on blood pressure. Firstly, it increases the releases of hormones such as adrenaline that encourage the constriction of blood vessels, making them narrower and increasing the pressure in them. Secondly, caffeine makes us more edgy. This can make us react more powerfully to life's stresses and strains, which can in turn cause our blood pressure to creep up.

Increase omega 3 intake
These vital fatty acids that I champion so often are essential for virtually every system in the body, including high blood pressure. They are metabolized to form prostaglandins, which play many regulatory roles. There are many types of prostaglandins, but the ones that are formed from omega 3 help relax the muscular walls of blood vessels, assisting in widening them. They also help reduce inflammation, which over the years can not only damage the inner lining of blood vessels, but can also make them less flexible.

Key ingredients:
Low sodium/high potassium salt—helps reduce the damaging effects of sodium on blood pressure
Bananas—rich source of potassium
Grapes—contain two compounds that help widen blood vessels
Spinach—rich source of potassium
Lentils—rich source of potassium
Chili—vasodilator (widens blood vessels)
Salmon—rich in omega 3
Red beets—packed with nitrates that increase nitric oxide, which helps widen blood vessels

Recommended recipes:
Spicy coconut dal, page 88
Whole wheat bean quesadillas, page 112
Red beet, red onion, and goat cheese tart, page 130
Immune-boosting jumbo shrimp curry, page 134
Broiled mackerel fillet with sautéed fennel and leek, page 137
Mackerel marinated with red beets and horseradish, page 140

D DIGESTIVE SYSTEM

BLOATING

Bloating is a common, but rather subjective experience; most people describe it as feeling very full, with a tightness in the abdomen, and often physical swelling too. It is caused by gas in the digestive tract, which is produced by our gut bacteria. This happens when the gut bacteria begin to ferment certain components of our food. Different foods may be problematic for different individuals, but it's often foods with a natural sugar content, such as fruit or starchy carbohydrates. Some sugars can also feed bad bacteria in the gut, which can make bloating worse, as can constipation.

Eat herbs to reduce gas
Some foods have a track record for reducing gas and easing bloating, often plants with strong aromas, like many herbs. The chemicals responsible for the pungent aromas and flavors can often break down and disperse gas. Many can also relax the gut wall, and even regulate movement of gut contents. Great examples are peppermint, fennel, caraway, aniseed, and basil.

Stay hydrated to avoid constipation
As odd as it sounds, being dehydrated can exacerbate bloating. We need sufficient water (about 6–8 glasses a day) to ensure that fiber will swell up in the digestive tract and help keep the bowels moving. If we become slightly constipated, stools stay in the bowel for longer and fermentation can occur. Lovely! Staying regular is vital, and hydration is an important part of that.

Encourage good gut bacteria
The "good" bacteria in our digestive tract regulate almost every aspect of digestion, from breaking down foods, to manufacturing nutrients, even maintaining and repairing intestinal tissue. Even the slightest imbalance or weakening of this bacterial community can cause problems. Less desirable bacteria can begin to flourish, and these are very often the ones that cause gas and bloating when trigger foods are eaten. Many people find that improving their gut flora can work miracles. There are several ways to do this: the first is to consume probiotic foods, such as high-quality live probiotic yogurt. The other is to eat prebiotic foods, which are rich in compounds that act as a food source for the good bacteria, causing them to grow and flourish. This includes onions, parsnips, Jerusalem artichokes, sweet potatoes, and more. A word of warning, though: the first few times you eat prebiotic foods, you may get more bloated and gassy at first. Sit this out, as it's a normal response and will quickly pass if you give it a chance.

Keep a symptom diary
Although not strictly a dietary intervention, keeping a symptom diary is vital. Log your symptoms, along with what you ate and drank, every day for a few weeks. You may start to see certain patterns forming, and notice that certain foods or beverages are more problematic for you than others, and you can then start to avoid them.

Key ingredients:
Mint—breaks down gas and relaxes the gut wall, giving rapid relief from bloating
Aniseed, basil, caraway, fennel—break down and remove gas
Live probiotic yogurt—packed with probiotic bacteria to help support your body's own bacterial colony
Jerusalem artichokes, parsnips, sweet potatoes—powerful prebiotics that encourage growth of good bacteria
Papaya—contains an enzyme called papain, which may help ease bloating
High-fiber foods (legumes, whole grains)—help keep you regular, reducing the risk of bloating

Recommended recipes:
Probiotic layer crunch, page 34
The digestive dynamo, page 47
Tomato and lentil soup, page 54
Baked sweet potatoes with omega hummus, page 110
Vegetable crumble with cheesy oat topping, page 123
Chickpea and sweet potato beta bake, page 126
Tummy tea, page 160

CONSTIPATION

Constipation is one of the most common non-serious health concerns in the Western world. The real problem comes when it turns into a chronic, long-term issue, which is sadly on the increase. The most common factors are lack of fiber in the diet and insufficient water intake. Fiber swells up and stretches the gut walls, which contain special receptors that sense this stretching. The muscles in the gut wall then contract in a series of waves known as peristalsis, the constant, natural, rhythmical movement that keeps us regular. For it to take place we need enough fiber, and to take in enough fluid to allow the fiber to swell. Stress, some medications and insufficient physical activity can also cause or worsen constipation.

Eat more fiber
Increasing fiber is really a case of switching to whole foods and reducing your intake of processed foods such as ready meals and carbohydrates like white bread, white rice, and white pasta. Instead, eat more fruit, vegetables, nuts, seeds, legumes, and grains. If you like rice, choose brown; if you like bread, choose multigrain.

Stay hydrated
Drinking enough water will make sure that the fiber in your diet swells up and stimulates peristalsis, keeping things moving along nicely.

Key ingredients:
Apples—packed with a soluble fiber called pectin, which helps soften stools
Fresh fruit & vegetables—high in good-quality fiber, not to mention a vast array of micronutrients
Beans & pulses—a great source of fiber
Brown rice, oats—fiber-rich, low-GI grains
Dates—contain beta glucan, great for keeping things moving

Recommended recipes:
Blast-off breakfast bars, page 32
Kick-starter kedgeree, page 44
Garlicky white beans with kale and Parmesan, page 84
Apple and cinnamon oat squares, page 94

CROHN'S DISEASE

Crohn's disease is a chronic inflammatory disease of the digestive tract, causing a thickening of the gut walls and reduced functioning, which can result in symptoms from malabsorption of nutrients, to abdominal cramps, diarrhea, weight loss, fatigue, bloating, and even fever and joint pain. The exact cause is not known, but is believed to be autoimmune in origin: the immune system creates antibodies that attack the tissues in the digestive tract. Nobody knows why, but there are theories that it may be linked to viruses, certain foods, and even environmental factors. As with all conditions, it's best to place dietary management alongside medical treatment.

Eat the rainbow to increase antioxidants
Antioxidants are crucial for reducing inflammation, especially in surfaces they come into direct contact with, such as the digestive tract. Some of the inflammatory response is caused by free radicals, highly reactive, damaging compounds produced in the body. Antioxidants can buffer their effects and help reduce the severity of inflammation, as well as protecting tissues from long-term damage. Increase your intake of brightly colored fruits and vegetables such as red peppers, sweet potatoes, radishes, and red beets. The compounds that give them their bright colors are powerful antioxidants.

Increase omega 3 to manage inflammation
Different fats provide different actions in the body. Increasing our intake of omega-3 fatty acids from sources such as oily fish and flax seeds helps the body produce more anti-inflammatory compounds,

which can drastically and rapidly ease inflammation. We can also reduce our intake of omega-6 fatty acids and arachidonic acid, found in red meat and vegetable oils, which can accelerate inflammation. A Mediterranean-style diet, rich in oily fish, olive oil, vegetables, and fruits, provides an optimal balance.

Eat less raw food

I usually encourage people to eat more raw fruit and vegetables where possible. However, a lot of evidence shows that this can be problematic in Crohn's disease, as it can be quite hard work for the digestive system, which is fine in a healthy person, and can improve digestive function. However, with Crohn's the bowel needs to be rested, especially during episodes of flare-up. Soups, stews, and well-cooked vegetable dishes are ideal.

Encourage good bacteria

The evidence about probiotics in Crohn's disease is mixed, but I think they are beneficial for several reasons. Firstly, good bacteria in the gut improve digestion in general, which can only be a good thing. Secondly, these bacteria play a role in repairing and maintaining the lining of the gut, which can be beneficial for Crohn's sufferers. We now know that the gut bacteria help regulate the immune system, both locally and systemically, which may explain why some clinical trials have shown that patients with better gut flora have fewer relapses of their condition. I recommend a good-quality live probiotic yogurt, and perhaps a good-quality probiotic supplement of some kind.

Key ingredients:

Red peppers—antioxidant rich
Sweet potatoes—antioxidant rich
Oily fish (salmon, mackerel, herring)—packed with anti-inflammatory omega 3
Live probiotic yogurt—rich in good bacteria

Recommended recipes:

Asparagus and smoked salmon egg dippers, page 42
Thai fish soup, page 50
The beta booster, page 86
Baked sweet potatoes with omega hummus, page 110
Red beet and pea risotto with mint and feta, page 124

HEMORRHOIDS

Hemorrhoids are distorted blood vessels in the lower bowel and anus. They arise most commonly from persistent constipation, or straining during bowel movements. Either way, there is increased pressure on the blood vessels in the lower bowel. This causes them to become distorted, and for sections of them to bulge out and to bleed.

Increase fiber intake

This may be stating the obvious, but many people take in incredibly small amounts of fiber on a daily basis. Fiber from fruit, vegetables, whole grains, legumes, and so on will soften the stool, making it easier to pass. It also helps bulk up the stool, which in turn stimulates stretch receptors in the gut wall. This increases contraction of the gut walls, which moves gut contents along more effectively, helping to relieve constipation.

Stay hydrated

The second part of the picture is to stay hydrated. Sufficient water intake will cause dietary fiber to swell. This swelling allows the stimulation of stretch receptors. Aim for a good 6–8 glasses of water per day.

Eat flavonoid-rich foods

Flavonoids have been widely studied in recent years, and have even made it into conventional pharmaceuticals. They are known to strengthen the blood vessel walls, therefore helping make them more resilient to damage and distortion. They're found in foods including blueberries, chocolate, red wine, and red peppers, among others.

Key ingredients:

Oats—rich in soluble and insoluble fiber to maintain regularity
Brown rice, quinoa—other fiber-rich staples
Berries—packed to the hilt with vessel-protecting flavonoids
Red onions—another flavonoid-rich food

Recommended recipes:

Probiotic layer crunch, page 34
Purple power salad, page 78
Apple and cinnamon oat squares, page 94
Goodnight spiced cherry crumble, page 146

IRRITABLE BOWEL SYNDROME (IBS)

IBS is one of the most common digestive complaints. It can manifest as constipation, diarrhea, bloating, gas, digestive cramps, and urgency to go to the bathroom, either in isolation or in combination. The symptoms often come and go, and many sufferers experience periods free of symptoms and periods with regular attacks. For many people, the symptoms will arise after eating.

Diarrhea IBS: avoid insoluble fiber
There is evidence to suggest that those who suffer from IBS characterized mostly by diarrhea may benefit from reducing the amount of insoluble fiber they consume. This is found in foods like bran, whole grain bread and cereals, and beans and other legumes.

Constipation IBS: increase soluble fiber
Soluble fiber swells up in the digestive tract and actually softens the stool. This increases the size and bulk of the stool, which stretches the gut wall. There are stretch receptors in the gut wall, and once activated these cause a reflex contraction of the muscle walls in the gut. This causes a natural rhythmical contraction in the gut called peristalsis, which moves gut contents along. It is also important to stay hydrated. Drinking enough water (6–8 glasses per day) is vital to allow soluble fiber to swell in the digestive tract and offer the benefits described.

Strengthen gut flora
Gut flora, the "good bacteria" that live in our digestive tract, are involved in regulating almost every aspect of digestive health. They have shown great benefit in issues like bloating, diarrhea, and constipation, so encouraging them is of obvious benefit to sufferers of IBS.

Key ingredients:
Oats, dates—rich in a soluble fiber called beta glucan
Brown rice, beans & other legumes—good sources of fiber
Apples—rich in a soluble fiber called pectin
Fresh herbs—all known to ease bloating and gas
Live probiotic yogurt—helps top up good bacteria

Recommended recipes:
Apple and cinnamon oat squares, page 94
Vegetable crumble with cheesy oat topping, page 123
Baked eggplant with tomato and lentil stuffing, page 129
Pineapple papaya and mint frozen yogurt, page 145
Probiotic mango smoothie, page 158
Tummy tea, page 160

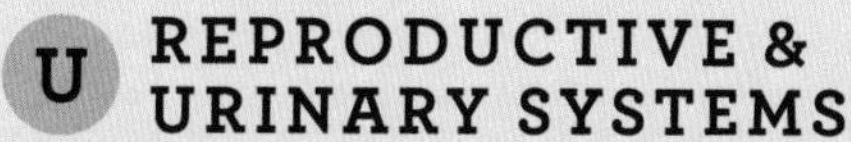

REPRODUCTIVE & URINARY SYSTEMS

CYSTITIS

Cystitis is usually caused by bacterial infection in the bladder and urinary tract, often by E. coli, the bug commonly associated with food poisoning. This lives naturally in certain areas of the genito-urinary and digestive tracts. If it finds itself in areas where it wouldn't normally be, it can cause infection by embedding itself in the walls of the urethra and bladder. The immune system moves in to deal with the invaders, and as a result the walls of the bladder and urethra become inflamed, which is what causes the pain and discomfort that most people experience during cystitis.

Consume cranberries
Cranberries and cranberry juice have a longstanding reputation as a remedy for cystitis, and it seems there is some truth in it. Cranberries contain a compound that is thought to pluck *E. coli* from the walls of the urinary tract, and also prevent attachment. It seems to be better for prevention than treatment, but many people do claim to get relief from cranberry juice during an attack.

Stay hydrated
One of the best ways to clear cystitis is by drinking plenty of water, thereby increasing the amount of friction against the urinary tract wall as the urine moves through it, which can help dislodge the bacteria.

Key ingredients:
Cranberries—stop bacteria sticking to the urinary tract walls
Celery—increases urinary output

Recommended recipe:
Cranberry and celery blast, page 162

ENDOMETRIOSIS

Endometriosis involves endometrial tissue, which usually lines the womb, growing in areas outside the womb, which could be anywhere within the pelvic cavity. This rogue endometrial tissue will behave in exactly the same way as that found in the womb; in other words it will respond to hormonal signals throughout the menstrual cycle, and will grow and bleed in the same way as the regular womb lining. This can cause pain and swelling. The exact causes are unknown, but conventional treatment usually includes hormonal therapies such as differing varieties of the contraceptive pill, and sometimes anti-inflammatories.

Increase phytoestrogen intake

These are compounds found in plant foods that are chemically similar in shape to the estrogen made in the body, which means they can naturally bind to estrogen receptors. This gives them potential benefit in managing hormone-related issues. They are found abundantly in legumes such as chickpeas, fermented soy foods like miso and natto, and even ingredients as humble as rhubarb.

Increase omega 3 intake

These vital fatty acids can help to take the edge off some of the pain during a flare-up of endometriosis. This is because omega 3 helps the body create its own natural anti-inflammatory compounds.

Key ingredients:

Chickpeas—high in phytoestrogens
Fermented soy products—fresh miso, natto, and tempeh are all rich sources of phytoestrogens
Oily fish (salmon, mackerel, trout, herring)—packed with omega-3 fatty acids.

Recommended recipes:

Edamame and chickpea salad with lime, chili pepper, and cilantro, page 61
Sesame soy salmon and vegetables with coconut rice, page 120
Chickpea and sweet potato beta bake, page 126

MENOPAUSE

Menopause comes about when the ovaries stop working properly and the levels of the hormones they normally release begin to fluctuate as they become less effective as each cycle continues. When this happens, the brain starts to release other hormones that usually activate certain processes within the ovaries, in an attempt to resuscitate them. The effect of these hormones, plus a drop in hormones like estrogen that would normally be released by the ovaries, causes chaos in the body, and many symptoms arise from this.

Eat foods rich in phytoestrogens

These are naturally occurring plant chemicals that are very similar in shape to the body's own estrogen. As such, these compounds can bind to cells in tissues that are responsive to estrogen. Some of the symptoms that arise in menopause are caused by the fact that these tissues have suddenly had their estrogen supply cut off, so they go crazy like a kid that has been denied candy. It is thought that phytoestrogens deliver their effect because they can bind to the receptors that are crying out for estrogen. This fools them into thinking that there is adequate estrogen present and stops them from making such a fuss.

Increase bone-building nutrients

One of the big issues that arises from estrogen decline is a loss of bone density, so it is vital to supply your body with the nutrients it needs to maintain bone density. While everyone focuses on calcium, it is actually rather difficult to not get enough calcium in your daily diet, unless you are have a very unusual diet. Taking in yet more calcium could actually be harmful to the kidneys and even the heart in the long term. I like to use the analogy of bricks on a building site. While the bricks are indeed the structural material that everything is made out of, without a team of builders, nothing will happen. The bricks will just sit there. The same applies to bone health. We need to focus on the nutrients that are involved in the absorption, transport, and utilization of calcium (the big ones are vitamin D and magnesium), while of course keeping the calcium-rich foods coming in too. This way you not only provide the nutrients that make up the structural material of the skeleton, you also supply what it needs to do its work.

Eat oily fish every day

Firstly, these will help you with bone health in light of what is mentioned above. However, the omega-3 fatty acids can help with hot flashes too. Omega 3 is metabolized into several different communication compounds in the body, including a group of chemicals called prostaglandins. One of the roles that these chemicals play is to regulate the circulatory system, and they may well help reduce excessive dilation of the blood vessels, which leads to hot flashes. The omega-3 fatty acids are also incredibly useful for elevating mood and easing the symptoms of depression and anxiety, so can be a powerful tool if you find that menopause is affecting your moods.

Control blood sugar

Two major issues in menopause are mood swings and bouts of low energy. While hormonal changes are responsible, a few simple dietary changes can help to take the edge off them. The key is following a low-GI diet. This means eating foods that release their energy very slowly and steadily, drip-feeding the blood sugar and keeping it nicely even and stable. Foods such as whole grains, lightly cooked vegetables, lean proteins, and dairy products are top of the list, and refined carbohydrates like white bread, white rice, and white pasta are banned! To take this a stage further, try to ensure that you have a good-quality protein and good-quality carbohydrate together at each meal. When you combine ingredients in this way, the meal will take longer to digest, longer to release its energy, and be much more gentle on your blood sugar levels.

Key ingredients:
Mackerel—packed with calcium, vitamin D and omega-3 fatty acids
Brown rice —low GI and packed with energy-giving B vitamins
Miso—bursting with phytoestrogens
Chickpeas—packed with phytoestrogens
Flax seeds—packed with phytoestrogens and omega-3 fatty acids

Recommended recipes:
Kick-starter kedgeree, page 44
Edamame and chickpea salad with lime, chili pepper, and cilantro, page 61
Edamame dip with chili pepper and garlic, page 76
Baked salmon with herbed omega crust, page 132

PERIODS, PROBLEMATIC

Many women suffer from hormonal problems, especially issues such as dysmenorrhea (heavy, painful, and problematic periods). There are many possible reasons for this, from increasing stress levels, to environmental pollutants and even overuse of the contraceptive pill. Infections can also create these types of problems. Although the cause is highly unlikely to be related directly to nutrition, changing your diet can most certainly help to reduce some of the symptoms.

Eat plenty of essential fatty acids

Eat plenty of foods like almonds, avocados, and most importantly of all, oily fish. The essential fatty acids they contain, such as omega 3 and DGLA, can have a double-whammy benefit. DGLA from foods such as avocados and almonds helps regulate certain reproductive hormones, and can also reduce the production of compounds that cause contraction of the uterus (one of the big causes of menstrual pain). Omega-3 fatty acids such as EPA and DHA have a potent anti-inflammatory activity, so they can ease the pain and inflammation.

Eat the rainbow

Sadly, this doesn't mean brightly colored candies! I am referring to richly colored fruit and vegetables, such as bell peppers, red beets, sweet potatoes, and kale. Many of the compounds responsible for the bright colors in foods also have antioxidant and anti-inflammatory activity.

Increase vitamin C intake

This will help you absorb more iron from your food. One of the big issues for people with heavy menstruation, is loss of iron through bleeding. Vitamin C helps iron to be absorbed more effectively.

Key ingredients:
Mackerel—packed with omega 3
Salmon—very rich source of EPA and DHA
Almonds—rich in GLA/DGLA
Bright vegetables —rich in antioxidants
Spinach—rich in vitamin C and iron; eat it with tomatoes to enhance iron absorption

Recommended recipes:
Thai fish soup, page 50
Walnut and watercress salad with blue cheese, page 69
Stress-free smoked mackerel pâté, page 92
Broiled mackerel fillet with sautéed fennel and leek, page 137

POLYCYSTIC OVARY SYNDROME (PCOS)

PCOS is characterized by the formation of cysts on the ovaries, which are eggs that haven't formed properly. When an egg forms in the ovary, it eventually pops out of the ovary through the skin on the outside of it, and enters the fallopian tube, leaving behind a small sack of scar tissue within the ovary, which then secretes hormones that regulate different aspects of the menstrual cycle. In PCOS, the egg is unable to break free from the ovary, and instead forms a cystic bulge. The ovaries make more of the male hormone group, androgens. This causes symptoms such as facial hair growth, menstrual abnormalities, acne, and weight gain.

Eat a low-GI diet

There is a big link between insulin resistance and PCOS. Insulin resistance is a condition in which our cells are no longer responsive to the signals that insulin sends (see page 170). The role of insulin is to tell cells to take up sugar when our blood sugar rises following a meal, and when this system goes wrong there can be several negative consequences. Of these, the most relevant to PCOS is that the body secretes more and more insulin to try and compensate for the cells' lack of responsiveness. Insulin spikes cause the ovaries to manufacture higher levels than normal of the male hormones, the androgens, specifically testosterone. This makes the walls of the ovaries much thicker, preventing the egg from breaking out, thus causing cysts to form.

The best way to start getting insulin sensitivity in check is to eat a low-GI diet, which will stabilize and even out blood sugar. It means consuming things that release their energy slowly, drip-feeding blood sugar levels. When sugar is released at a much more even pace, it won't be necessary to fire out such huge surges of insulin. In time, this will make our cells much more sensitive to insulin, reversing some of the insulin resistance. Low-GI foods include whole grains such as brown rice, brown pasta, quinoa, and bulgur wheat, lean proteins, such as oily fish and poultry, and lightly cooked vegetables. To create low-GI meals, use these ingredients, and make sure you include a good-quality protein, a good-quality carbohydrate, and ideally a good-quality fat source in each meal. In time, this approach can greatly reduce insulin resistance.

Eat oily fish
How did you know I was going to say that? The physiological importance of the omega-3 fatty acids lends them well to almost any health challenge. In PCOS there are bouts of inflammation in reproductive tissues, especially at different stages of the cycle. Omega-3 fatty acids help your body create its own, natural anti-inflammatory compounds.

Eat phytoestrogen-rich foods
Although the scientific data are mixed, anecdotal reports suggest that phytoestrogen-rich foods can be helpful in PCOS, and may help balance out hormones.

Key ingredients:
Brown rice, quinoa, bulgur wheat—low-GI
Mackerel—high omega 3, good-quality protein for making low-GI dishes
Salmon—high omega 3, good-quality protein for making low-GI dishes
Miso—phytoestrogen rich
Chickpeas—high in phytoestrogens

Recommended recipes:
Kick-starter kedgeree, page 44
Edamame and chickpea salad with lime, chili pepper, and cilantro, page 61
Tuna steaks with sweet potato wedges and greens, page 118
Chickpea and sweet potato beta bake, page 126
Salmon and jumbo shrimp skewers with citrus quinoa salad, page 142

PROSTATE HEALTH

The male prostate gland goes through several growth cycles during its lifetime. It starts at around 1 gram in weight at birth and grows to around 18 grams in a fully grown adult. However, from around age 50 onward, many men experience another growth cycle and begin to experience inconvenient symptoms linked to prostate enlargement. The prostate begins to enlarge when levels of the hormone testosterone drop in relation to levels of estrogen. When this occurs, testosterone's super-strength cousin dihydrotestosterone (DHT), becomes more active, and stimulates the growth of prostatic tissue. This normal growth, known as benign prostatic hyperplasia (BPH) is mostly harmless, but in some circumstances this can set the stage for prostate cancer.

Eat lycopene-rich foods
Lycopene is a carotenoid that displays a deep red color in plants, and is the compound responsible for making tomatoes red. It is believed to reduce the risk of BPH progressing into prostatic cancer. The exact modes of action are not clear, and some evidence also shows little benefit. However, most available evidence to date does show benefit and populations that have the highest tomato intakes showed lower levels of prostate cancer and BPH. Some studies of lycopene supplements have shown reduced markers of prostate cancer in participants taking lycopene.

Increase beta sitosterol
There is strong evidence that this plant-derived fat reduces symptoms associated with enlarged prostatic tissue. The evidence is so strong that in some parts of Europe they have been used in prescription drugs. How it works isn't exactly clear, but it is thought to reduce swelling, and it certainly seems to reduce the size.

Eat more zinc-rich foods
Zinc is a vital mineral for the normal day-to-day functioning of the prostate. Although there is no evidence to suggest that zinc can treat prostate problems, supporting the overall health of this gland is of obvious benefit.

Key ingredients:
Tomatoes—the richest source of lycopene
Almonds—packed with beta sitosterol
Pumpkin seeds—packed with beta-sitosterol and zinc
Avocados—rich in beta-sitosterol
Shrimp—a good source of zinc

Recommended recipes:
Gazpacho, page 58
Roasted vegetable and guacamole open sandwich, page 62
Immune-boosting jumbo shrimp curry, page 134

WELL-BEING

As well as helping with individual conditions, many nutrients can also provide an all-around boost for the body, helping it to function more effectively. Here are some more general well-being issues that diet can help.

HANGOVER

Those all-too-familiar symptoms can hit hard! Most of them arise from dehydration and depleted minerals and water-soluble nutrients like B vitamins and vitamin C.

Increase magnesium intake
Some hangover symptoms are believed to be related to magnesium depletion. Green leafy vegetables are among the best sources of this vital mineral.

Top off your electrolytes
These are lost in abundance during a drinking session, and are vital for maintaining water balance and the functioning of every cell. Add a pinch of good-quality sea salt to every glass of water you drink in the morning.

Top off B vitamins
The B vitamins are water-soluble and can be depleted easily when we drink a lot of alcohol because our urinary output goes up, leaving us lethargic and fuzzy-headed.

Key ingredients:
Green leafy vegetables—packed with magnesium
Eggs—B vitamins and magnesium
Sea salt—contains important electrolyte minerals
Whole grain bread—full of B vitamins and magnesium

Recommended recipes:
Easy eggs florentine, page 38
Spinach, tomato, and shiitake mushrooms on toast, page 40
Wake-up juice, page 158

FATIGUE

A little bit of fatigue is perfectly normal, but some of us seem to be in a state of near-constant tiredness. Thankfully, many of the factors that have been linked to increased fatigue are within our control. Poor diet, not dealing with stress effectively, and insufficient exercise all contribute. Whatever the cause, there are dietary steps you can take to start feeling better fairly quickly.

Eat a low-GI diet
One of the fastest ways to zap your energy is to experience frequent blood sugar swings. Foods that release their energy rapidly, such as refined carbohydrates, cause our blood sugar to rise sharply, and what goes up must come down. Blood sugar levels are tightly controlled, and when we experience surges we secrete the hormone insulin, which tells the cells in the body to take up more sugar. The more insulin released, the more rapidly the glucose is taken up. Blood sugar levels then plummet and we feel tired and sluggish. Most of us then reach for another "pick-me-up" snack, and the whole process starts again. The key is to choose foods that will release energy slowly, and to combine them to slow this down even more. Start by choosing whole grain, complex carbohydrates such as whole wheat breads and quinoa, fresh vegetables, and lean proteins such as oily fish. The next thing is to combine them. Try to have a complex carbohydrate, lean protein, a vegetable, and plenty of good fats with every meal.

Increase B vitamin intake
The B vitamins are among the most commonly deficient nutrients, but are vital for energy production. They are abundant in many foods, but are easily destroyed in cooking and processing, and we can easily not take in enough. When glucose enters our cells, it has to be converted into a substance called ATP, which is what our cells actually run on. The B vitamins don't exactly "give" you energy, but are directly involved in several stages of this conversion process. They are abundant in whole grains, yeast, mushrooms, and asparagus.

Eat little and often
It is better to eat small meals every couple of hours, instead of three big meals a day, or indeed skipping meals. Eating every couple of hours will keep your blood sugar levels topped off and the nutrients coming in!

Stay hydrated
Even slight dehydration can really deplete your energy levels. Try to drink 6–8 glasses of water a day.

Key ingredients:
Lean proteins (fish, poultry, eggs, tofu)
Brown rice—B vitamins, a low-GI carbohydrate source
Quinoa—rich in protein and complex carbohydrates, a low-GI-grain alternative, and full of B vitamins
Green, leafy vegetables—full of B vitamins and magnesium

Recommended recipes:
Spinach and feta scramble, page 31
Kick-starter kedgeree, page 44
Energy bombs, page 96
Banana-peanut oat bars, page 98
Salmon and jumbo shrimp skewers with citrus quinoa salad, page 142

INDEX

FURTHER READING

JOINTS & BONES

The Academy of Nutrition and Dietetic's (formerly known as the American Dietetic Asssociation) "Understanding Osteoporosis" on **http://www.eatright.org/Public/content.aspx?idd=5550**

METABOLIC SYSTEM

The Academy of Nutrition and Dietetics "Diabetes" on
http://www.eatright.org/Public/list.aspx?TaxID=6442452078
The American Diabetes Asssociation's "Food" on
http://www.diabetes.org/food-and-fitness/?loc=GlobalNavFF

MENTAL HEALTH & NERVOUS SYSTEM

A fantastic and comprehensive website by Dr. Alex Richardson and Professor Michael Crawford from Oxford University: **http://www.fabresearch.org/**
The Brain Bio center also has a good research database that can be found here:
http://www.foodforthebrain.org/content.asp?id_Content=488

HEART & CIRCULATION

The Academy of Nutrition and Dietetics' "Heart and Cardiovascular" on
http://www.eatright.org/Public/list.aspx?TaxID=6442452082
The American Heart Association's "Nutrition Center" page on
http://www.heart.org/HEARTORG/GettingHealthy/NutritionCenter/Nutrition-center_UCM_001188_SubHomePage.jsp

REPRODUCTIVE & URINARY SYSTEMS

The National Cancer Institute's sectoin on Prostate Cancer
http://www.cancer.gov/cancertopics/types/prostate
Information from Prostate Cancer UK on links between diet and managing prostate issues:
http://prostatecanceruk.org/information/living-with-prostate-cancer/diet-and-prostate-cancer
A huge wealth of data on diet and prostate issues:
http://www.prostate.org.au/articleLive/pages/Diet-and-Prostate-Cancer.html

In his first major cookbook, TV's Medicinal Chef and nutrition expert Dale Pinnock presents his unique approach to cooking and health. Many seemingly humble ingredients—even chocolate—contain powerful phytonutrients that have been shown to have beneficial effects on a range of medical conditions. With 80 easy-to-make, tasty recipes, Dale shows how simple it is to incorporate them into your everyday diet, giving a boost to all the body's systems and improving energy levels.

With a glossary of key ingredients, advice on how your diet can make a real difference to thirty common ailments, and simple symbols to indicate which conditions each recipe can help, eating your way to good health has never been easier or more delicious.

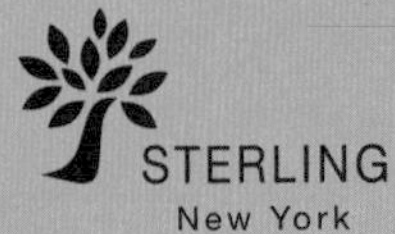

First Sterling edition 2013

First published in 2013 by Quadrille Publishing Limited

ISBN 978-1-4549-1049-7

Distributed in Canada by Sterling Publishing
c/o Canadian Manda Group, 165 Dufferin Street
Toronto, Ontario, Canada M6K 3H6

For information about custom editions, special sales, and premium and corporate purchases, please contact Sterling Special Sales at 800-805-5489 or specialsales@sterlingpublishing.com.

Manufactured in China

2 4 6 8 10 9 7 5 3 1

www.sterlingpublishing.com

Editorial director: Anne Furniss
Creative director: Helen Lewis
Project editor: Laura Gladwin
Art direction and design: Smith & Gilmour
Photography: Martin Poole
Food stylist: Lucy Williams
Props stylists: Wei Tang & Polly Webb-Wilson
Production: James Finan